PALEO
Cleanse

30 Days of Ancestral Eating to Detox, Drop Pounds,
Supercharge Your Health and Transition into a
Primal Lifestyle

Camilla Carboni
Melissa Van Dover

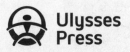

Ulysses
Press

Published in the U.S. by:
Ulysses Press
P.O. Box 3440
Berkeley, CA 94703
www.ulyssespress.com

ISBN13: 978-1-61243-392-9
Library of Congress Control Number: 2014943034

Printed in Canada by Marquis Book Printing Inc.

10 9 8 7 6 5 4 3 2 1

Acquisitions Editor: Kelly Reed
Managing Editor: Claire Chun
Editor: Renee Rutledge
Proofreader: Lauren Harrison
Index: Sayre Van Young
Front cover and interior design: what!design @ whatweb.com

Distributed by Publishers Group West

NOTE TO READERS: This book has been written and published strictly for informational and educational purposes only. It is not intended to serve as medical advice or to be any form of medical treatment. You should always consult with your physician before altering or changing any aspect of your medical treatment. Do not stop or change any prescription medications without the guidance and advice of your physician. Any use of the information in this book is made on the reader's good judgment and is the reader's sole responsibility. This book is not intended to diagnose or treat any medical condition and is not a substitute for a physician.

To our loved ones for your ongoing support and encouragement, to our readers and to the world—may this contribute to good health and your best life.

Contents

PART 1

THE PALEO FACTOR

Introduction: Our Stories

About a year and a half ago, we each were tackling a full-time job in marketing, as well as a night and weekend commitment to writing. This left little time to focus on our health and well-being. Time slipped away from us and later that year, determined to get back on track with daily exercising, we took on the extreme home workout DVD the *Insanity Workout* in full force and rocked it!

Doing *Insanity* nightly meant eating a lot—a lot of protein and carbohydrates in particular. It was awesomely delicious and a great excuse to consume as much lean meat as possible. The diet centered around a hearty bagel breakfast, whey protein shakes, amino energy drinks, smoked salmon, and steak salad wraps. We couldn't eat enough.

When the nine weeks of *Insanity* finally ended, we were exhausted and somewhat satisfied. Don't get this wrong—we love the *Insanity* workout and still do *Insanity* regularly today, only the diet we were consuming left us both feeling depleted and experiencing regular blood sugar lows. It wasn't a good enough diet to consider continuing long term, but we didn't realize why just yet.

It wasn't until Camilla's boyfriend, Matt, bought a copy of *The Paleo Manifesto* by John Durant—which explained exactly why wheat, dairy, and the legume family should be avoided—that it all started to make sense to us.

Less than a month later, we began our 30-Day Paleo Cleanse, which focused on eating as much lean meat, fruit, and vegetables as possible, while exercising regularly and writing about it, of course. That Cleanse laid the foundation for this book.

Camilla's Story

I grew up in a very close middle-class family that knew the importance of diet, exercise, and general well-being. Mealtimes were family times, and we all lent a helping hand as we prepared delicious, balanced meals. We didn't eat out often; we avoided fast food, processed foods, and candy. We were certainly healthier than most people we knew in South Africa, and I believe South Africans to be pretty healthy in general.

After a very difficult and emotionally taxing two-year struggle, my dad lost his battle against bone marrow failure. The news came a week before my sixth birthday. My mother and I were forced to regain some sense of normality in our lives, but naturally something was always missing. Together we made it work. We had mother-daughter TV nights, painted, cooked homemade pizza, devoured chicken soup, and baked what I still believe to be the most delicious chocolate cakes in the entire world.

I became an avid figure skater and competed in the young woman's section for my province. I was fit and toned, yet I still had troubled skin and got severe tonsillitis very regularly. For someone who exercised so much and ate well (or so I thought) we couldn't quite figure out the problem. I was presented with a whole range of topical "solutions" and strong antibiotics. Nothing worked. We finally came to the conclusion that there was something else at play and that all these medicines were doing were trying to treat the symptoms, rather than the root cause.

About six months later I found myself in the waiting room of a well-known Ayurvedic doctor (a form of alternative medicine based on the science of life) who had trained with the reputable Deepak Chopra. I had broken my ankle figure skating and had unknowingly skated on it for many months as I was trained to withstand pain. Subsequently, I had worn away the tissue surrounding the bone and tendon in my right foot. This Ayurvedic idea was a last resort. I had tried physiotherapy and acupuncture at the top sports medicine clinic in my city, had x-rays, had worn a removable boot cast for six weeks, and had still not seen any sign of improvement on the x-rays or in day-to-day mobility. Plus I was still in pain, though I didn't regularly admit it, as I desperately wanted to return to the skating rink.

The doctor greeted me kindly and, unlike a regular physician, did not begin with "What brings you in?" Instead he asked to feel my pulse and gestured for my wrist. I was baffled but obliged and sat in silence for about a minute while he appeared to be concentrating very hard as he listened to my pulse. Finally he looked up at me and said that I was too stressed out (that comes with the territory of a Type A personality, doesn't it?), that I needed to cut out wheat, dairy, brown rice, and lentils from my diet, and that I needed to rebuild the tissue around the tendons that support my right ankle. I'm not too sure how he picked all that up from my pulse, but a couple of moments later I was lying on the massage bed and he was applying steam to my broken ankle while massaging it vigorously with a proprietary sesame oil blend. Who was I to judge? I'd tried Western medicine for months without any luck.

When he finally spoke it made sense to me. It all came back to treating the root cause. The steam and pressure on the area forced the cells to focus on the depleted tissue, ultimately speeding up the recovery process. It was a little wacky, and the opposite of the "apply ice" theory in Western medicine, but truthfully, it made sense.

He wanted me to come in once a week for steam treatments for about two months, after which he said I'd be back to my former strong self. I asked him when he thought I may be able to return to figure skating and his answer was astounding:

"You can go right now," he said. And so I did.

My ankle has never been a problem since. I also gave up cheese, yogurt, brown rice, and lentils. I did this for about seven years and felt better. I had far more energy and far less congestion and allergy complications. It was clear to me that not only can disease be brought about by a "dis-ease" in the mind (we can think ourselves sick, just as we can think ourselves healthy), but disease can also manifest from a dis-ease in the body.

But then came university and all went rapidly downhill. I took an additional major, leaving little time for working out, not that there was an ice rink in my university town anyway. Plus, the numerous late nights left me turning to carbohydrates and energy drinks like the majority of college students do, which caused a vicious cycle of bad health.

In 2006 I visited America for the first time. I went on a student exchange program to the University of Iowa. I had the time of my life, but one thing I cannot erase from my mind is the extent of fast food, frozen food, and preservatives consumed by American college students.

I remember sending a photograph of a vending machine in the lobby of my residence that had burgers sitting in it for days. My friends back home in South Africa were mortified. There were TV dinners on the shelves that didn't require refrigeration. I had to wipe the oil off my pizza and my roommate couldn't believe that I had never eaten deep-fried onion rings. Worst of all was the cafeteria, which was an all-you-can-eat buffet of waffles, Sloppy Joes, pizza, and sugary cereals for a very nominal fee. I was horrified by the sheer gluttony of the industrial food buffet and only ate there once. Finding healthy options became more of a challenge than ever before.

Later that year I returned to South Africa, and now, more aware than ever before, began to return to stricter Ayurvedic eating habits while I completed my thesis. I kept this up whenever and wherever possible, spending only $15 CAD a week on food when I moved to Vancouver to work and save for my U.S. immigration. People cannot believe it when I tell them this, but honestly, I ate well. My main diet consisted of beef-stuffed butternut squash, sushi, and green vegetables.

In early 2009, green card in hand, I packed my bags and moved to Hawaii. I sought sunshine, freedom, and translucent waters, but got more than I bargained for. For a year and a half I worked two jobs, lived in three different apartments, sipped many a tropical cocktail (until I realized that I was allergic to pineapple) and ate at happy hours whenever possible. You can't beat $5 appetizers!

In June of 2010 an account director of a renowned resort in Waikiki contacted me about one of my restaurant reviews on Examiner.com. Three months later I was working for the resort full-time. I worked hard and was committed to many evening events; I got to the beach very seldom and I ate daily at the hotel cafeteria (think comfort food buffet), like everyone else. I gained weight, experienced blood sugar spikes and lows, drank way too much coffee, and eventually realized I was lactase non-persistent.

When I turned 28 I came to the conclusion that while life was fabulous in Hawaii, it wasn't really suited to the life I was trying to live. I wanted to settle down in a place of my own, get healthy again, and truly live the American Dream. That's when my boyfriend, Matt, took the reins and convinced me to move to his home state, Colorado.

Two years later and here I am, living in my very own home in Colorado. Only Matt, despite understanding caloric intake and always keeping fit and lean, didn't share my thoughts and beliefs about being low-carb and dairy-free. We ate plenty of pizza and pasta, and not nearly enough vegetables. That was until recently when he came across *The Paleo Manifesto*, a book by John Durant that finally spoke to him in the language he understood and gave him the insight he needed to radically change his diet. I was ecstatic.

He read the oversized book in three days and on day four I found myself being dragged to a bookstore at a ridiculous hour for a Paleo recipe book. Interestingly, the recipe book even referred to the Ayurvedic diet.

Now that Matt was sold on a healthier diet idea, I wasn't about to miss a beat. A week later, along with Melissa we went fully Paleo, cold turkey. It tied together everything I'd learned and experienced over the years. Paleo simply made sense.

I then realized I wasn't suffering from my regular blood sugar roller coaster ride or migraine headaches, plus my skin cleared up entirely.

After a few weeks, neither of us had food cravings and my seasonal allergies began to diminish.

The better I felt the more I realized just how much of an effect wheat, dairy, and sugar have on the body. Healing yourself starts from the inside and we should all take note of what we are feeding our cells. I've never felt better. The rest is history. Now it's your turn to try.

Melissa's Story

When I was younger I didn't pay much attention to my health or wellness. Let's be honest, I was a kid in America, which basically sums it up. I was also stick thin and could eat whatever I wanted without gaining weight. I did sports occasionally, but outside of that I was pretty lazy. I, like most kids in the USA, liked TV *a lot*. I also managed to find every excuse to skip out on PE and since I was skinny, no one saw an issue with it. This taught me a lesson: Just because you're skinny doesn't mean you're healthy.

So let's fast-forward to when I was about 17 and everything began to change. I started to get sick; I was having random heart palpitations, becoming dizzy, and having trouble breathing. This is where my story really begins. I started a seven-year-long journey of sickness. When you're 17 and you start getting these symptoms, it's really not considered normal, and it shouldn't be. During the next four years I underwent every test known to man and "potentially" had every disease as well. I had to wear heart monitors; I had more blood drawn than I think was in my body; I had MRIs, ultrasounds, and the list goes on.

From what the doctors could tell, I had a high white blood count and my thyroid antibodies were through the roof. This resulted in me being told that I had leukemia, cancer, a heart murmur, an issue with my endocrine system, an infectious disease...and believe me, this was just the tip of the iceberg. Then, when they couldn't concretely figure anything out, I was considered crazy! I learned two things during this time: 1. Generally doctors in the United States only focus on diseases that are in their specialty, and 2. If a doctor doesn't know what you have, you're simply considered nuts.

Fast-forward two years. I'm in college. At this point I've been up and down with not feeling good. I'm still having the heart issues; in fact, I've been rushed to the ER because my heart rate jumped to 175 bpm and wouldn't come down. Believe me, being carried out of a dorm room on a stretcher at 1 a.m. is not a fun experience and since it was college, everyone saw. I spent the night in the ER, which was an experience. The nurses treated me horribly until they realized I wasn't some stupid college student with alcohol poisoning. While the nurses had warmed up to me when they decided I wasn't on drugs, the doctor didn't seemed to care that I was there and sent me home after six hours, telling me nothing was wrong with me even though my pulse was still at 130 bpm. *Yeah, because that is totally normal.*

After this experience a couple of things started to happen: 1. My symptoms began to change, and 2. I was in the ER every six months. Some of the other symptoms I started to get were focused around my GI system, and, overall, I was really, really tired. I was experiencing these symptoms almost every day and this continued for two years.

This is when I started to put it all together. Yes, you heard right. After the multiple doctors I had seen, *I* figured it out, with the help of my mother. Sometime during this period, my mother, who is a nurse practitioner, started asking if I noticed any trends with what I was eating. I didn't notice anything particularly with *what* I was eating, but I did notice that everything generally happened around *when* I was eating.

Finally I managed to figure it out on a family vacation to South America. I was in the town of Las Calientes at the foot of Machu Picchu, basically in the middle of nowhere. I had a Pisco Sour, a glorified margarita with foam on top. I got really sick after this; I was lucky that nothing serious happened. The foam on top of the drink was made out of egg whites. This is the point where I thought, okay, maybe I was allergic to egg.

A few months later when I got the flu shot this was confirmed. To say the least, I had quite an unpleasant reaction to it. I ended up going to an allergist and made them test me for eggs and, Bingo! I had found part of the problem. I cut out eggs cold turkey. Most of my symptoms went away and I started to feel better.

Over the next couple of years I was doing better. However, I was still tired overall and still had symptoms periodically. I noticed that they would get worse after I exercised heavily for a period of time; I later determined that this was because I increased the amount of wheat in my diet when I increased my exercise, but we'll get back to that.

I had given up on trying to go to doctors; honestly, I had had enough during the previous few years to last me a lifetime. Finally, I decided I'd give it one last chance. This was unfortunately during a time that I started to feel worse again. I was getting aches in the joints in my hand. I had a history of rheumatoid arthritis in my family, and since I already had one autoimmune disease that affected my thyroid, (Hashimoto's) I was nervous I might have another.

My ANA test, which is a general test for autoimmune diseases like lupus and rheumatoid arthritis, was about a hundredth of a point off from being positive.

At this time one of my good friends, who happened to have a lot of food allergies, recommended that I go to her doctor, who was both an allergist and an immunologist. This doctor looked at the whole picture, not just his specialty, and this is where things started to get interesting.

The doctor ended up running a battery of tests on me and discovered I had a few other food allergies. In particular, I was allergic to wheat. So not only did he direct me to cut those foods out, he also explained that certain foods could make autoimmune diseases worse, wheat and tomatoes being two examples. This research was also something I had read about in *The Paleo Diet* by Loren Cordain. My doctor's theory was that my allergies and immune system were feeding off of one another and giving me many of my symptoms. He believed a correction of my diet would help. His recommendation of a diet for me was essentially a Paleo Diet. Needless to say, if I continued on my current path, things were only going to get worse.

The biggest difference came when I cut out wheat. Essentially, all of my symptoms went away like a puff of smoke. I didn't have that weird malaise tiredness anymore and I had no stomach issues. Finally, after seven years I was back to normal. Back to normal may not seem that great, but it is if you haven't been there in a while. A few times I cracked and had wheat again. It wasn't a fun slope back down to where I had begun.

Then Camilla and I decided to take a Paleo pact: a 30-Day Paleo cleanse. I was on board even though we only decided to do it about a week before we started. It wasn't a lot of time to get ready, but we were committed and energized so we made it happen. It was the beginning of a healthier lifestyle, that focused on avoiding foods that aggravated my allergies and autoimmune disease prevention. To put it mildly, I'm feeling amazing now.

CHAPTER 1

What Is the Paleo Diet?

It began with *Hominins* about 2.6 million years ago, in the depths of jungles and the heat of grassy plains. The early *Hominins*—our ancestors—roamed freely, living off the earth and hunting for protein and animal fats to fuel their developing bodies. During the winter, the meats they consumed kept them warm, and throughout the summer, the fresh berries they picked gave them bursts of natural energy. They were an organic species, living harmoniously off the abundance that our earth provides and the prey that they outsmarted.

Over millions of years the diet they consumed remained consistent, yet seasonal, and reliant only upon that which nature provided. It nourished their cells, allowing them to evolve into *Homo sapiens*. As *Homo sapiens* they grew taller, stood upright on two feet, and began to entertain thought.

They were the predecessors to the species we have become. They lived solely off the land and spent their days chasing prey and wandering fields to gather fruits and vegetables to feed their families.

But here *we* are today. We seem to have forgotten our heritage. As humans we now live largely off genetically modified and overly processed substances and spend our days riding the elevators of office buildings before returning home to slouch on our sofas while devouring TV dinners and large sodas.

What Happened?

After 2.4 million years of roaming free—spanning a hundred thousand generations—our ancestors grew curious about cultivating food rather than searching and hunting for it. It seemed like a great idea (or so they thought), and just like that, Agriculture was born.

The birth of the Agricultural Era changed the way our ancestors lived and fueled their bodies. While their diet evolved, their genetics and natural dietary needs remained virtually unchanged.

The Agricultural Era adjustments meant that the typical daily activities of running miles on a hunt and wandering fields for fresh berries ceased to exist. These adjustments also led to a significant alteration of their diet—food by-products suddenly became a large part of daily consumption. Seeds and grains were introduced as a starch-based dietary supplement. This movement also encouraged the consumption of dairy, seizing the opportunity to "liberate" the natural milk from farm animals and drink it freely.

It all seemed like such a great idea. Starch was filling and cheap, and dairy was readily available. Both made for quick and accessible dietary "fixes" to keep nourished. The problem was, and still is, that the body is not naturally developed to digest these food by-products. So the rise of Agriculture simultaneously resulted in the downfall of the human diet.

When you do the math, the Agricultural Era began just over 12 thousand years ago, spanning less than five hundred generations and equating to only a fraction of the time that our species has existed (0.5 percent of the time, to be exact).

Extensive research has shown, and continues to illustrate, that our human species is not naturally tolerant of grain, dairy, or legumes. It also demonstrates that to gain optimum health, we should eat what we can easily absorb nutrients from. Our Paleolithic ancestors had it right; we should in fact be following their diet.

What Exactly Did Our Paleolithic Ancestors Eat?

They ate what the earth provided and what they could hunt. Their diet consisted largely of animal protein and vegetables, varying in quantity and ratio depending on the region and landscape that they called home. The category of animal protein included hunted game and wild-caught fish. Their vegetable intake consisted mainly of roots and tubers. They would also consume berries whenever available. Seeds and legumes (which include soybeans, chickpeas, and peanuts) were not regularly consumed. Both seeds and legumes are naturally designed by nature to propagate and therefore pass through the body virtually untouched. Consequently, seeds and legumes failed to provide our ancestors with the energy they sought in food and therefore served them little to no purpose. Back then, they ate to live, not the other way around.[1]

When Did the Paleo Diet Gain Popularity in Our Modern Era?

Back in the 1970s, evolutionary science placed its attention and consideration on the concept of returning to Ancestral eating habits in order to achieve optimum health. In 1975, gastroenterologist Walter L. Voegtlin published the book titled *The Stone Age Diet: Based on In-depth Studies of Human Ecology and the Diet of Man*. The book suggested that following a diet similar to our Paleolithic ancestors' would improve our health. This trend continued as various articles, books, and papers of the same theme surfaced throughout the 1980s and '90's.

In 2002 Loren Cordain introduced a book on the subject, *The Paleo Diet*. While the diet itself is nothing new—being that it's based on Ancestral eating—the popular book and Cordain's detailed findings made the world look twice. Cordain caused others to wonder if he was indeed right and if we had in fact drifted off of our natural dietary course. Cordain coined the term "Paleo Diet," after the Paleolithic Era. Call it what you will—the "Caveman Diet," the "Ancestral Diet," the "Primal Diet," the "Stone Age Diet," or, simply, the "Natural Human Diet"—it all refers to the diet that we are biologically adapted to eat.

Since the release of Cordain's book, the Paleo Diet has gained the attention of millions of curious, health-conscious *Homo sapiens* around the globe. In 2013 "Paleo Diet" was the most searched diet term on Google. This curiosity has led to more research into the accuracy of the Diet's foundation and to many more books on the subject, all aiming to illustrate the benefits we would gain in returning to our natural eating habits.

What Is Considered Paleo, and What Isn't?

It seems complex at first, but truthfully Paleo Diet food choices are very logical:

- Say "Yes!" to organic fruits and vegetables, nutritional nuts, fish, healthy fats, and grass-fed meats.
- Say "No way" to grains, dairy, refined sugar, vegetable oils, legumes (like peanuts, lentils, and chickpeas), industrial foods, GMOs (genetically modified organisms), preservatives, sodas, candy, and tons of salt.

It's not rocket science; just use common sense. The Golden Rule of the Paleo Diet is not to eat anything you know is not good for you. If you're unsure, give it the *Flintstone Test*: Would our ancestors (hunters, gatherers, cavemen) have been able to keep food on their cave "shelf" for months? No! Good-bye long-life foods and frozen dinners. Would cavemen have been able to bake donuts? No! Good-bye processed sweets and pastries. Would cavemen have been able to eat fresh meat and handpicked vegetables? Yes! Hello earth to table!

Now that you know the basics, let's go into the science behind why the Paleo Diet supports our natural biology.

Why Should I Say "Yes!" to Fruits, Vegetables, Healthy Fats, and Grass-Fed Meats?

Fruits: Fruits are typically rich in fiber and contain beneficial quantities of vitamins, antioxidants, and water. Fruits also contain phytonutrients, which are believed to promote cellular health and keep disease at bay.

Vegetables: Vegetables contain various vitamins, minerals, and antioxidants, depending on their variety. Many vegetables are also rich in natural fiber, which is vital to gastrointestinal function. All dietary schools generally agree that the nutrients found in vegetables are necessary to human health.

Healthy Fats: Healthy fats can be consumed in various forms, such as nuts, fish, grass-fed meat, and coconut oil. These foods are fatty in a good way—they provide your body with omega-3, vitamin E, and other fatty acids. These are all considered essential for brain and heart health, and are believed to aid the body in absorbing vitamins while preventing internal inflammation.

Grass-fed Meats: Grass-fed meats come from animals that have been fed their own natural diet. Consequently, those animals are less prone to disease and the food you consume is free of genetically modified grains and hormones that are toxic to your body.

Why Should I Say "No Way" to Grains, Dairy, Refined Sugar, Vegetable Oils, and Legumes?

Gluten: Gluten is found in wheat, a grain designed by nature to be untouched when digested so that it can return to the earth to propagate. The majority of wheat protein consists of gluten, which the body cannot absorb and causes internal inflammation when consumed.[2]

Grains: Grain has the same impact on the body as gluten (which also falls into the grain category but has become such a well-known term that we mention it as a freestanding topic). As with gluten, toxic proteins in grains such as corn and barley cause digestive complications in humans, as we are not designed to digest the food group.[3]

Dairy: Dairy products derived from animals were only introduced to our human digestive system during the Agricultural Era and are consequently not foods that we are naturally able to digest (with the exception of human breast milk during childhood). As a result, many people are unable to consume dairy, or are lactase non-persistent (commonly known as "lactose intolerant").[4]

Refined Sugar: Refined sugar is typically found in soda, candy, and other industrial foods. Too much sugar of any kind is damaging to our health as it causes insulin reactions and an excess of glycogen in the body. Excessive sugar intake can cause diseases such as diabetes, obesity, and gout, and is believed to accelerate aging.[5]

Vegetable Oils: Vegetable oils such as canola oil, soybean oil, and corn oil are all by-products that were introduced with the Agricultural Era. They contain grains and seeds that we now know have toxic proteins indigestible to humans. In addition to these toxins, vegetable oils have very high quantities of omega-6 fatty acids. A healthy human diet needs fatty acids, but excessive amounts of omega-6 prohibit the body from properly absorbing omega-3 fatty acids, the healthier fat.

An excess of omega-6 (which is easy to achieve since vegetable oils are present in the majority of industrial foods) continues to attribute to obesity, allergies, and cancer.[6]

Legumes: Legumes, like grains, contain proteins that are toxic to the human body. Because they are not able to be absorbed by our digestive system, and prevent us from absorbing the nutrients found in legumes, these toxic proteins are sometimes referred to as antinutrients. The consumption of legumes is essentially an empty calorie and one that inflames the gut.[7]

Now that we've delved into the dietary guidelines of the Paleo Diet, let's take a look at how this differs from the traditional Western diet.

CHAPTER 2

The Traditional Food Pyramid vs. the Paleo Food Pyramid

A Food Pyramid is a triangular-shaped diagram divided up into groups that represent the major food groups. Consumption of these food groups is suggested for optimum human health. The base of the Food Pyramid, the largest area of the shape, represents the group from which we are advised to consume the most foods or calories each day. Then, as the divisions move upward toward the vertex of the pyramid, the suggested quantities decrease, and the very top section is the food group with the smallest suggested intake.

The First Food Pyramid

The first Food Pyramid was established in Sweden in 1974[8]; it suggested that daily caloric intake should consist mainly of grain, starch, and dairy. The middle row of the Pyramid included vegetables, fruits, nuts and seeds, and the smallest suggested food group included protein (animal meats and fish).

Seventeen years later, in 1992, the United States Department of Agriculture (USDA) introduced the Food Pyramid we are most familiar with today. It looked like this:[9]

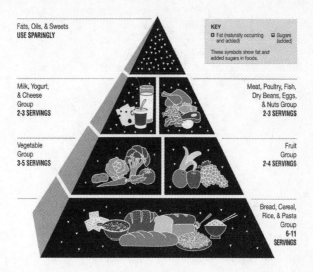

Despite a decade of additional research, grain and starch still formed the largest suggested food group. Dairy, however, was moved up closer to the top of the Pyramid, alongside protein. Vegetables and fruit were placed side by side in the second largest area of the Pyramid. The category of "Fats, Oils, and Sweets" formed the smallest category at the very top.

In 2005 that Food Pyramid was updated to adjust the suggested dietary intake ratios. The new diagram, called *MyPyramid*, portrayed a suggested balance between the intake of grains, vegetables, and dairy. This change coincided with the research paper "Dietary Guidelines for Americans" that promoted whole grains and dairy as equally essential to our diet as vegetables. Coincidently, this was also around the same time that the Milk Regulatory Equity Act of 2005 was lobbied for approval. It was passed in 2006 and increased milk prices across the nation.

Notably, *MyPyramid* adopted a slightly different layout and added the element of exercise, represented by the human figure climbing the stairs on the left-hand side of the Pyramid. This was certainly a welcome addition and a more well-rounded approach to health and well-being. That said, the recommended ratio of food groups remained concerning. The 2005 Food Pyramid looked like this:[10]

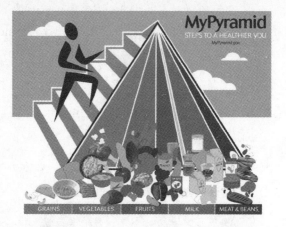

That Food Pyramid remained the standard for six years. In 2011 it was changed again to the new format of the Food Pyramid (although it's no longer in pyramid form), which is still current today. Below you will find that this latest version, *MyPlate,* clearly illustrates recommended serving sizes by food group:[11]

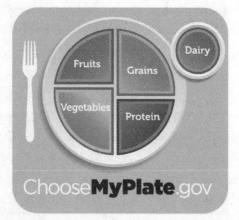

As you can see from the above illustration, grains and vegetables are tied in first place for equal importance in our diets, followed by a secondary balance of fruits and protein. Dairy follows just behind, with a marginally smaller intake suggestion, represented by the glass of milk on the top right. Fats and oils are no longer represented on the diagram.

It should come as no surprise that a typical Paleo Food Pyramid is quite significantly different from all the others we have examined. Let's take a look at our Paleo Food Pyramid example below and why it is so different.

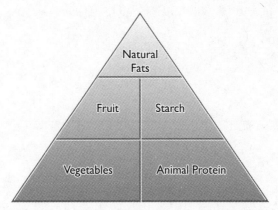

In the Paleo Food Pyramid, protein and vegetables claim the dominant spots, followed closely by fruits and healthy starches, and then by natural fats. Grains and dairy don't have a place in the Paleo Food Pyramid, and refined sugar products are not included either. It's almost like turning the traditional Food Pyramid on its head, but frankly, it's actually more tradition-based than the Swedish or USDA versions.

The Paleo Food Pyramid ties strongly to its Paleolithic roots. In Paleolithic times, protein and vegetables were the most readily available food sources and provided our ancestors with the majority of their daily nutrient intake. Picked fruit, healthy starch, and natural fats were their next source of consumption. These natural fats were a vital component to their health, providing omega-3 fatty acids, which contributed to the development of the human brain. Grains, legumes, and sugar were neither easily digestible nor as accessible as they are today. For 2.5 million years, these foods were simply not a part of our Ancestral Diet, and they remain unnatural to us today. Our bodies have simply not evolved to process these foods.

Our modern-day eating style is a whole lot more complex than it needs to be. The thousands of product choices we find on our grocery store shelves and the sheer variety of alternatives available in each food group have complicated things and created more confusion than benefit. In reality, our optimal diet consists of clean, uncomplicated foods that are natural, unprocessed, and seasonally accessible.

CHAPTER 3

Marketing Myths Debunked

After receiving thousands of mixed messages on what "healthy" means, most of us are totally confused. When we look at the Food Pyramid as we did in the previous chapter, it's hardly a surprise. We see it in action every day. People reach in droves for 2 percent milk, oatmeal packets, and diet foods. The multibillion dollar health industry is influential and strategic, attempting (very successfully thus far) to convince us of what we need to eat and what we should avoid in order to be healthy. The push toward whole grains and dairy consumption are perfect examples of heavily funded advertising campaigns. Another example is the "low fat" enterprise, which has drawn about as much attention as the Hallmark-sponsored Valentine's Day holiday. The fear of cholesterol and the calorie-counting epidemic are other examples, and we can go on for days. The fact is we've all been inundated with marketing messages that have overtaken our common sense and clouded our vision, preventing us from doing the research we should have done many years ago.

It's time to start thinking very seriously about what your own health is worth. It's time to start acknowledging health messages for what they really are—excellent examples of persuasive marketing—

and then research the facts and determine what is truly best for your personal health.

Is the consumption of dairy, grain, and genetically modified crops benefiting your health or contributing to your medical expenses?

Good marketers make their product sound even better than it is. That's their job. It's your job to see marketing for what it is and then make your own decisions.

Spotlight on GMOs

The Agricultural Industry has expert marketers working for them. Monsanto, for example, spends millions of dollars advertising their product each year. What exactly is their product? Monsanto is a leading producer of genetically engineered (GE) seed. The company was the first in the world to genetically modify plant cells (this occurred in 1982, just one generation ago) and to plant fields of genetically modified crops. Yes, that falls under the "No way" GMO category!

Monsanto's GE seeds are used to produce large quantities of vegetable oil and corn, soybean, and wheat products—the ones we find at our local grocery stores cleverly disguised in almost all of the industrial, pre-packaged food. Monsanto also produces pesticides from toxic glyphosate and has sold and acquired numerous spin-off companies, including artificial sweetener brands.

In the past years, much debate has surrounded Monsanto's marketing and methods, with fears and concerns largely focused on the nutritional integrity and future of Agricultural growth.[13]

Recently, Monsanto spent over $5 million fighting the latest initiative to place GMO labels on all products.

Are Whole Grains Really Healthy?

GMOs pose an obvious concern, but what about whole grains? While whole grains do have nutritional contents, such as fiber, iron, and magnesium, these nutrients cannot be readily absorbed by our bodies. As already discussed, seeds are naturally formed to stay intact in order to propagate. When digesting grains, the body attempts to remove the toxins they present, activating an immune alert to clean out the intestines. During this self-cleansing process, the intestines become inflamed, which causes damage to the intestinal lining and can result in leaky gut.[15]

The more we consume foods that cause our bodies to self-cleanse, the more at risk we are of "leaky gut" symptoms. The simplest way to understand leaky gut is to think of a protective barrier that is designed to keep toxins out, but that has been punctured, enabling tiny undesirable particles (such as bacteria, viruses, and undigested food) to seep through. These particles are then transported through the body, and the immune system has no choice but to attack them. Once your intestinal wall or "gut" wall is compromised, you are at risk of a number of side effects, including bloating, stomach cramps, skin irritations, and fatigue. When unwanted particles make their way to the bloodstream, allergic reactions can also worsen. Grain, particularly with the presence of gluten and a diet high in refined sugar (which stimulates the growth of yeast), has been shown to be the strongest cause of leaky gut.

What about Refined Grains?

If you are going to eat any grain, white rice is actually the least toxic. Yes, we are aware that brown rice has been made to appear as the healthier option, but this is just an example of what marketing has led us to believe. Brown rice does have higher nutrient quantities of fiber, iron, and magnesium; however, it has a much higher quantity of phytic acid as well. Phytic acid is a saturated cyclic acid that stores phosphorous in many plants, most notably in bran and seeds. Phytic acid is not digestible by humans, and it prevents the absorption of minerals, such as zinc, iron, magnesium, and calcium. White rice, on the other hand, is stripped to the bran during processing, which rids the white rice of phytic acid, leaving it to consist almost entirely of carbohydrates. Therefore, while brown rice technically has a higher nutrient content than white rice, those nutrients are not available to be absorbed by the body and instead place us at risk of leaky gut.[16]

What's the Scoop on Dairy?

The dairy industry (driven by the Milk Processor Education Program, or MilkPEP) spends millions on advertising each year. Over the past two decades MilkPEP has paid celebrities top dollars to be photographed with milk on their upper lips as part of the widespread "Got Milk?" campaign you are no doubt familiar with. While we were writing this book, MilkPEP announced that they will be retiring their "Got Milk?" campaign for a new initiative, titled "Milk Life." The CEO of MilkPEP told reporters that they plan to spend $50 million on the "Milk Life" campaign to promote the "nutritional value of milk."[17]

Don't Be Fooled

Marketing is always at work. Industry misconceptions are increasingly common. We are presented with so many, often conflicting, messages about health that it becomes problematic to determine what is actually the truth and what is just a marketing tactic. We've heard it all: the rise and fall of soy; ongoing debates over meat products; the protein scare of veganism; the grain, dairy, and refined-sugar battle; calorie-counting low-fat diets; "quick-fix" detoxes; and other latest fads. It's no wonder we're left so utterly confused with no clear idea of how to begin regaining our former, Ancestral health.

What's more, the cost of not knowing is becoming more and more expensive. Each year in the U.S. alone, we spend over $140 billion on obesity-related conditions, and that doesn't include the cost of cancer treatments, which can be tied to inflammation within the body.[18] As

David J. Getoff says in the documentary *The Perfect Human Diet*, "Health is not convenient, but it's not half as inconvenient as a fatal illness."

So we ask you—what's your health worth? We think the billions of dollars at question should be invested in your personal well-being. It's time to revisit the way things were before we began suffering from modern day diseases. It's time to explore the benefits of the Paleo lifestyle.

CHAPTER 4

Benefits of the Paleo Lifestyle

Many people mistakenly label the Paleo Diet as a mere detox or fad diet. While we recommend you transition into Paleo eating with the Cleanse outlined in this book, it is far more than just a 30-day commitment, and the benefits you will no doubt experience will justify why that is. The Paleo Diet is a way of eating that began with our ancestors and which supports our natural digestive functions. It's not a quick fix or a craze—it's a lifestyle.

We began our Paleo journey by doing a 30-Day Cleanse and it worked wonders for us, which is why we transitioned into the Paleo lifestyle full-time. It's also why we were inspired to share our journey with you. We hope this experience will be as beneficial for you as it was for us. The more people that discover the power behind Paleo eating and the incredible transformation it has on the body, the more the Paleo Diet becomes a common lifestyle.

The below benefits, among others, may become noticeable while living a Paleo lifestyle. Let's examine each of these in a little more detail.

Bodily Changes

Reduced Inflammation: In Chapter 1 we covered the effects of grains, legumes, refined sugar, vegetable oils, and dairy on the body and how these foods irritate our digestive system, causing inflammation and worsening autoimmune diseases. The toxic proteins found in grains, the high amount of omega-6 found in legumes and vegetable oils, the excess of glucose and fructose in refined sugar, and the hormones found in dairy all have an adverse effect in and on our body. Sticking to Paleo-friendly foods can assist anyone suffering from certain specific autoimmune diseases and any other inflammatory issues. Simply put, most Paleo-friendly foods do not cause aggravation within the body and therefore enable our organs to function as designed.[19]

Superior Physical Performance: You've no doubt heard that a sizeable consumption of carbohydrates is necessary for peak athletic performance, particularly endurance. The fact is the body actually performs better when fueled by healthy fats. Why is this so? Because when the body can easily digest the food it's being fed, it can more efficiently convert food into energy.[20] Over the years, many professional athletes have discovered this truth and turned to a Paleo lifestyle to enhance their careers. The Los Angeles Lakers basketball team is a great example of a group of well-known professionals who practice Paleo for improved athletic performance. The growing CrossFit movement is another excellent example of this trend.

So Long, Roller Coaster: It's become a very common and accepted notion to experience blood sugar highs and lows, post-lunch lulls, and mood swings after eating. The thing is, food-induced roller-coaster rides aren't normal; and by that, we have to clarify that the roller-coaster ride isn't normal *if* you eat foods that you are meant to have. Since the Paleo Diet steers you clear of all those foods your body is not naturally accustomed to, you will suddenly find yourself with a consistent blood sugar level. Don't worry—while roller-coasters are fun, being on level ground is a good thing when it comes to health.[21]

Clearer Sinuses: Sinus complications often result from infection and allergy problems. The eradication of dairy and the elimination of grains on the Paleo Diet mean that our organs, glands, and mucous membranes are free of food-aggravated irritation and inflammation. When our body is inflamed, our internal fluids that should move without interruption are restricted. Blockages can amount to serious infection and can often interfere with our ability to breathe clearly. If we simply reduce our intake of foods that cause or worsen inflammation and mucous buildup, we can prevent sinus complications before they happen.[22]

Adieu, Acne: Toward the end of the Cleanse we noticed that both of us had clearer skin. Overall we just looked healthier. While it's hard to explain exactly what it was that made us look healthier, it had a significant effect on our self-confidence. We were walking examples of the saying, "When you look good, you feel good." Plus, the best part was that people noticed and started to ask us what we had changed.

In 2002 Loren Cordain published an academic paper titled "Acne Vulgaris: A Disease of Western Civilization." At the time, the notion of acne stemming from dietary choices was generally disregarded, but the paper illustrated something interesting—that acne appeared to be a problem of the Western world, a direct connection to our Western diet that is heavily centered around grains, dairy, vegetable oils, and refined sugar. Those Western foods block our pores and sebaceous glands, which is caused largely by the hormonal change that consuming unnatural foods has on our body. Over 40 million Americans suffer from acne, and in 2004, the cost of acne-associated treatments in the U.S. exceeded $2.2 billion.[23] Understanding this side effect of Western eating can enable us to eliminate our acne by cleansing our body from within.

Adios, Headaches: About the same time that our mental clarity improved, Camilla noticed that she was not experiencing her normal migraines. She used to have migraines every week or so, and while she can look back now and see that they were in fact decreasing from the very beginning of the Cleanse, it was only after a few weeks that she realized they had completely gone away.

If you have ever suffered from headaches you will know all too well just how unpleasant they are. About 25 million Americans are said to suffer from migraine headaches.[24] That's a whole lot of miserable, unproductive people who are reaching over the counter for the likes of Excedrin and placing millions of dollars in the bank accounts of pharmaceutical companies each year. By merely eliminating many of the major food allergens, including wheat, dairy, and migraine-stimulating food products like MSG, aspartame, food coloring, and other artificial additives, which the Paleo Diet does, we can come a long way to curing headaches naturally.[25]

Weight Loss: The end of our 30-Day Paleo Cleanse was probably the most dramatic in terms of physical change. We each saw a decrease in body fat percentage. Additionally, we each experienced weight loss. This weight loss occurred without an increase in our normal exercise level. While exercise is extremely important, one's diet can have just as large (if not more) of an impact on weight loss.

Mental Changes

Sharper Mental Clarity: Mental clarity was a huge benefit for each of us. Often throughout the day we had trouble focusing; we both experienced this and figured it was the "norm." However, we noticed roughly two weeks into the Cleanse that we were able to concentrate better and for longer periods of time on the Paleo Diet. This particular benefit has been huge for us.

A good night's sleep, regular exercise, healthy eating to control blood sugar levels, and an adequate intake of nutrients are all welcome side effects of the Paleo Diet. These side effects support brain health and aid mental clarity. High quantities of sugar and carbohydrates are the culprits that send our blood sugar levels on a roller-coaster ride, clouding our vision and befuddling our mind. These items are almost entirely eradicated on the Paleo Diet, and thus, mental clarity is improved.[26]

Good-bye, Cravings: It's not your fault that you're craving sugar, bread, and pasta. They are addictive. Say what?! Yes—refined sugar, bread, and pasta all include opioid peptides, which are opiates, and are related to the likes of opium and heroin. One of the best changes we experienced was the disappearance of our cravings for Paleo-unfriendly foods, like bread and candy. During the initial few days we had several cravings for sugar and wheat; interestingly enough, this started to subside shortly after getting them out of our systems. Toward the end of our Cleanse these cravings were essentially gone.

When you cut addictive foods out of your diet, as you will on the Paleo Diet, you will experience a short period of withdrawal, during which you will continue to crave those foods. Once your willpower conquers your cravings and you resist temptation for just a few days, your blood sugar levels will begin to stabilize and your body will return to its natural, consistent state.

Less Stress: Stress can be brought upon by many reasons, but lack of sleep, sugar crashes, and food cravings are generally major contributors. On the Paleo Diet you are consuming foods that your body can easily digest and which don't require the body to attack itself in order to break down unwanted food particles. When food particles go where they are meant to, digestion is efficient, resulting in normal levels of insulin and acid. As a result you will notice a balance occur within your body. When your body normalizes, food-induced mood fluctuations diminish, resulting in the increased ability to manage stress.[30]

Overall Well-Being

Sounder Sleep: On the Paleo Diet, the disrupters of sleep almost entirely subside and a new, natural cycle results: Normalized blood sugar levels mean healthy, uninflamed organs, enabling restful sleep, which reduces stress and improves our ability to focus and maintain good health, in turn contributing to a sounder night's sleep. Snoring, which is a common sleep disrupter (for both yourself and your significant other) is another factor lessened by a Paleo Diet. By eating natural foods that can be easily digested, we reduce internal inflammation, which can be a common cause of snoring. *Shhhhhh*, don't tell the 12 million people in the U.S. alone suffering from disrupted sleep.[27] Just kidding, please help us spread the word about what appears to be the best kept secret of our time. We have become far too reliant on quick fixes and pill popping to eliminate our symptoms when the way to really cure the root cause is from within.

Mitigate Autoimmune Disease: It just so happens that particular autoimmune diseases can be aggravated by the consumption of Paleo-unfriendly foods. Research indicates that roughly 23 million-plus people in America suffer from autoimmune diseases.[28] Not so coincidently, autoimmune-exasperating food groups, such as grains that contain gluten, account for the largest daily caloric intake of most Americans. The removal of gluten from the diets of individuals who have celiac disease can help relieve their symptoms. Additionally, it is not unheard of that some individuals who suffer from autoimmune diseases realize relief from their symptoms when refraining from particular food groups.[29]

Stronger Immune System: Our immune system works hard to protect us against pathogens: viruses, bacteria, and other infectious agents. By consuming a typical Western diet high in refined sugar, grains, and legumes, we add to the body's workload, forcing our intestinal cells to cleanse themselves from the toxic proteins and high insulin dosage. This damages the intestinal lining, irritates the gut, and disturbs our natural equilibrium of probiotics, leading to immune system dysfunction. When the body expends a lot of energy counteracting internal inflammation, it has less energy to fight outside pathogens. Moreover, pathogens thrive in glucose-rich environments. Sticking to Paleo-friendly foods ensures the body is fed what it needs to operate naturally. It is then in peak health and best able to protect itself against bacteria. Nourishing your body with healthy Paleo foods is like providing your cells with the strength and armor they need to fight disease.[31]

Food as Medicine

All of the above—reduced inflammation, superior physical performance, blood sugar stabilization, clearer sinuses, clear skin, headache relief, sharper mental clarity, diminished cravings, sounder sleep, autoimmune improvement, reduced stress, and increased immunity—have everything to do with the fact that the Paleo Diet stabilizes one's metabolism, enables the body to more efficiently digest food, and allows the body to focus on being healthy. When you eliminate digestive complications and feed your body with the nutrients it needs, your organs function optimally, your intestines are not inflamed, and your cells flourish, flushing out toxins and keeping disease at bay.

The exact opposite has been occurring since we've introduced grains, dairy, and legumes into our diet. The inability to properly digest these foods and the subsequent harm this has on the body has resulted in "mismatch diseases." Leading Harvard evolutionary biologist Dr. Daniel Lieberman uses the term "mismatch disease" to explain the modern-day health issues that have festered from the fact that our Paleolithic bodies are poorly adapted to our modern-day diet and lifestyle.[32] It comes down to that simple saying: "We are what we eat."

Feed our bodies junk food and they will look and act like junk. Feed our bodies the nutrients we are naturally attuned to and we will look our best and function optimally. "Mismatch diseases" are the result of the human species going off course. We can correct our course, but to do so we must first correct our diet.

The idea of food as medicine is an ancient philosophy. In 431 BC Hippocrates said so eloquently, "Let food by thy medicine and medicine be thy food." Today, the concept of food as medicine is gaining popularity in our modern world, and the Paleo lifestyle is a perfect example of returning to ancient, natural eating habits to fuel our bodies with the foods they can draw nutrients from and consequently thrive off of.

By eating a diet of natural, unprocessed, chemical-free, and hormone-free foods, we are feeding our cells well and directly contributing to our own long-term health and well-being. What we choose to place in our bodies today has an enormous impact on how our bodies treat us today, tomorrow, and in the long-term future. We urge you to think about what you are eating. Choose well, eat well, and you will live well.

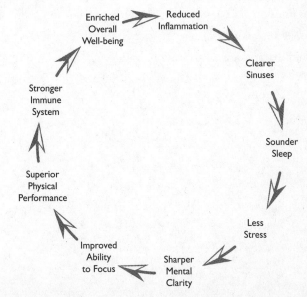

Putting It All Together

It is important to remember that the body and mind are one. Treat your body well and your mind will stay alert and, in turn, keep your body healthy. Diet and lifestyle are critical in overall well-being, and each aspect directly impacts everything else, both mentally and physically.

The diagram on page 41 serves to solidify the cyclic notion of our health, illustrating how a healthy diet promotes overall well-being.

PART 2

---///---

PREPARING FOR THE PALEO CLEANSE

CHAPTER 5

Your Journey to Health

"The greatest wealth is health."
~Virgil

There is a reason you hold this book in your hands today. Whatever it is that has led you to this point—to the start of your Paleo Cleanse— and whatever you seek to achieve on this journey, is yours to experience and to tell.

We hope this guide will provide you with the support and necessary resources to complete your Paleo Cleanse successfully. The following section includes a checklist that we recommend completing both before you start and after you complete your Cleanse. Filling out these worksheets will help you paint a clearer picture of exactly how you and your body have benefited from the Paleo Cleanse.

Your health is your most precious commodity. Let's prepare for your journey to health right now!

Pre-Cleanse Checklist

Measurements

Weight: _____lb. or kg   Waist: _____ in. or cm

Body Fat: _____ %   Hips: _____ in. or cm

Body Mass Index (BMI): _____   Biceps: _____ in. or cm

Water Mass Index: _____ %   Thigh: _____ in. or cm

Ailments

❑ Acne   ❑ Headaches

❑ After-Meal Heaviness   ❑ High Blood Pressure

❑ After-Meal Tiredness   ❑ High Cholesterol

❑ Allergies   ❑ Insomnia

❑ Asthma   ❑ Migraines

❑ Blood Sugar Spikes   ❑ Mood Swings

❑ Cramps   ❑ Overweight

❑ Diabetes   ❑ Skin Irritation

❑ Difficulty Waking   ❑ Sleep Apnea

❑ Exhaustion   ❑ Upset Stomach

❑ Food Cravings   ❑ Other: _____

Exercise Regimen

Average number of days per week you exercise: _____ days

Average number of hours per week you exercise: _____ hours

Types of Exercise (check all that apply and provide a brief description):

❑ Strength Training: _____

❑ Cardiovascular Training: _____

❑ Interval Training: _____

❑ Other: _____

General Energy Level

❑ 1   ❑ 2   ❑ 3   ❑ 4   ❑ 5
(Very Low)   (Below Normal)   (Normal)   (Decent)   (High)

Post-Cleanse Checklist

Measurements

Weight: _____lb. or kg   Waist: _____ in. or cm

Body Fat: _____ %   Hips: _____ in. or cm

Body Mass Index (BMI): _____   Biceps: _____ in. or cm

Water Mass Index: _____ %   Thigh: _____ in. or cm

Ailments

❑ Acne   ❑ Headaches

❑ After-Meal Heaviness   ❑ High Blood Pressure

❑ After-Meal Tiredness   ❑ High Cholesterol

❑ Allergies   ❑ Insomnia

❑ Asthma   ❑ Migraines

❑ Blood Sugar Spikes   ❑ Mood Swings

❑ Cramps   ❑ Overweight

❑ Diabetes   ❑ Skin Irritation

❑ Difficulty Waking   ❑ Sleep Apnea

❑ Exhaustion   ❑ Upset Stomach

❑ Food Cravings   ❑ Other: _____

Exercise Regimen

Average number of days per week you exercise: _____ days

Average number of hours per week you exercise: _____ hours

Types of Exercise (check all that apply and provide a brief description):

❑ Strength Training: _____

❑ Cardiovascular Training: _____

❑ Interval Training: _____

❑ Other: _____

General Energy Level

❑ 1	❑ 2	❑ 3	❑ 4	❑ 5
(Very Low)	(Below Normal)	(Normal)	(Decent)	(High)

CHAPTER 6

What Is the Paleo Cleanse?

Designed to get your health on track easily and enjoyably, and tailored for optimum impact based on our own 30-Day Cleanse experience, we bring you the easiest possible guide to getting started on your Paleo journey, or to revisiting a Paleo lifestyle.

Cleansing is considered to be vital to human health. It's only natural to overindulge at times and eat things we know we really shouldn't. We've all done it, so don't feel guilty—instead feel great about the journey you're about to embark on.

From time to time our bodies need to be given the opportunity to rejuvenate. Cleanses enable our bodies to purge, regenerate, and restore. The Paleo Cleanse might be considered the most natural cleanse there is.

Why You Chose Well

Of all cleanses, the Paleo Cleanse is most closely aligned with Ancestral dietary choices. It's like returning your body to its roots and nourishing it with the foods it truly needs.

In addition to the health benefits of returning to Ancestral eating, avoiding grains, dairy, the legume family, and refined sugar to eradicate toxins and clean the digestive tract, the Paleo Cleanse is unique (and desirable) in its inclusion of healthy fats, animal proteins, and dietary balance.

Unlike juice cleanses, soup cleanses, and supplement cleanses, the Paleo Cleanse is designed to refuel your cells through natural nourishment, not depletion. We are not going to ask you to starve yourself!

The Paleo Cleanse

The Paleo Cleanse is a 30-day introduction to the Paleo Diet. It is a month-long plan designed to be simple to follow, yet highly effective. It's just enough time to give you a taste of what the Paleo Diet can do for your body and your life.

To ensure you gain the optimal benefit after just 30 days, the Paleo Cleanse takes a stricter stance on the Paleo Diet than what is popularly followed. There are a number of different schools of Paleo thought that vary slightly in their approach to certain foods, such as grass-fed cheese and white potatoes. The stricter schools of Paleo do not permit such items, while others believe that if you introduce them into your diet without noticing adverse side effects, you may eat such foods in moderation without complications. Most schools of Paleo agree, however, that the best way to begin the lifestyle is by adhering to a strict Paleo Diet for at least the first few weeks. Only after that is the introduction of other food products to that base diet recommended. You can consider the Paleo Cleanse as your base Paleo Diet.

In Chapter 8 we will walk you through a complete list of Paleo-friendly food and foods you should avoid at all costs. We will also outline the foods that are Paleo-friendly, but that we recommend restricting at first, or at least during the 30 days of the Paleo Cleanse. Restricting these particular foods will accelerate your detox.

While you do not need to deprive yourself of nourishment on the Paleo Diet, we do advise watching your portion sizes and paying attention to your eating habits during the Paleo Cleanse month. We suggest this because your stomach stretches based on food quantity and because eating times are typically driven by blood sugar crashes and cravings. At first, your old habits may try to persist. Pay close attention to when you are eating and why, for you may just find that as your body adjusts to the new diet, your desired portion sizes and habits change as well. We also recommend granting yourself permission to go to bed when you feel tired and sleep in until your body naturally awakens you. We know that this is not a realistic practice for every day, but try to do this on your days off or when at all possible. As your body is rejuvenated by the Paleo Cleanse foods, it will begin to function differently. Try to let this Cleanse process be as organic as possible; let your body tell you what it needs. You might be surprised at how well your body functions when it's nourished with foods that support it rather than deplete it.

From the Paleo Cleanse to the Traditional Paleo Diet

While on the Paleo Cleanse, we suggest staying away from Paleo-friendly flours (such as coconut flour and almond flour), Paleo-friendly sugars (such as coconut palm sugar), all dairy (even grass-fed butter), and all alcohol. We also suggest restricting your consumption of nuts, oils, natural fats (such as avocado and animal fats), Paleo-friendly starches (such as yams and sweet potatoes), and fruits that contain high contents of fructose (such as bananas, melon, grapes, apricots, and papaya).

After the 30-Day Paleo Cleanse we recommend introducing these Paleo-friendly foods into your diet slowly. At that point your body will be detoxed, regenerated, and ready to take on an increased amount of healthy fats, starches, and natural sugars. That's when we'll have fun sharing Paleo dessert recipes with you.

The Paleo Cleanse Mantra

There is very little you need to remember as you begin your Cleanse journey. We've outlined everything you need in the chapters that follow and are always available to answer any questions you may have on our website: ThePaleoPact.com.

Before we begin walking you through preparations for the Paleo Cleanse in the following chapters, we encourage you to commit to living the Paleo mantra. The Paleo Cleanse is only fully effective if you follow a pure, Ancestral, lifestyle-based, environmental, and organic philosophy:

P ure: Foods that have no artificial properties.

A ncestral: Foods that our species is adapted to eat.

L ifestyle-based: Not a fad-diet, a way of life.

E nvironmental: Living off our earth and supporting it.

O rganic: The way nature intended.

It all comes back to choosing well, eating well, and consequently living well.

CHAPTER 7

How the Cleanse Is Set Up

The Paleo Cleanse is set up in a simple-to-follow formula. The Cleanse itself will last a total of 30 days, or roughly four weeks. You'll also need about a week to prepare. Before your Cleanse, you'll learn about the three categories of Paleo foods, perform a "pantry purification," and purchase the *Paleo Cleanse Essentials* that you'll need. Then, for each week of the Paleo Cleanse, you'll be provided with a customizable *Meal Plan* and *Grocery List*. The *Meal Plans* are crafted to transition your body into the Paleo lifestyle; however, unlike a normal cleanse, you'll actually be able to eat. Go food!

Each week we'll provide you with basic Paleo recipes that you will easily master and can later adjust to fit your specific taste buds. It will provide you with a solid foundation for living the Paleo lifestyle and will cleanse your system, helping you to lose body fat and gain energy. Additionally, you'll be provided with our tips from each week. We detail what changes to expect both mentally and physically during your Cleanse, as well as the tips we've found that will help make your life easier.

Following the fifth week we'll provide you with a simple guide for transitioning into the Paleo lifestyle full-time, if you choose to do so. Luckily for you, at this point you will have done the heavy lifting, so transitioning to full-time will be a breeze. We'll also provide some resources for continuing your Paleo journey.

Here's to your successful Paleo Cleanse! Now let's get started.

CHAPTER 8

To Eat or Not to Eat

The categories of food that you need to be aware of while completing your Paleo Cleanse are: *Cleanse Foods, All You Can Eat, Paleo in Moderation,* and *Foods to Avoid at All Costs.*

The *Cleanse Foods* category contains the food groups that are included in the Cleanse *Meal Plan* choices. We suggest following the recommended quantities specified in each recipe.

The *All You Can Eat* category is the list of Paleo-friendly foods from which you can consume as much as you want. We say go for it, and don't worry about holding back! This category is nutritious and perfect for consumption during the Cleanse.

The third category, *Paleo in Moderation,* is a list of Paleo-friendly foods that we recommend you consume in moderation during the Cleanse. Yes, these foods are delicious and very much Paleo, but if your intention is to lose weight during your Cleanse and really clean out your system, you're going to want to restrict your intake of these food items.

The final category, *Foods to Avoid at All Costs,* are foods that are not considered Paleo-friendly. These foods do not adhere to the common Paleo Diet principles and you should avoid them both during your Cleanse and after, if you choose to transition into a Paleo lifestyle.

Cleanse Foods

Colorful Vegetables: Each color of the vegetable spectrum provides unique health benefits due to their mineral and vitamin contents. We need all the nutrients, so eat all the vegetables!

Fresh Fruits (low sugar content): Fruits are a natural source of fiber, potassium, and vitamin C. During the Cleanse, feel free to indulge in the low-sugar variety (i.e., apples, oranges, grapefruit, pears, and berries).

Eggs: Eggs are rich in antioxidants, iron, phosphorous, selenium, and various vitamins.

Coconut Oil: The coconut provides a healthy source of saturated fat and is slow to oxidize. This means you can turn up the heat and the oil contents remain unchanged and harmless to your body.

Olive Oil: Olive oil is a great option for dressing foods, such as salads, on the Paleo Diet. Note, however, that olive oil should not be heated as, unlike coconut oil, it has a high oxidization rate and becomes toxic at high temperatures. Olive oil eaten cold is great for your heart.

Avocado Oil: Avocado oil is a great option for cooking on the Paleo diet. It doesn't have the heavy flavor of coconut oil, so for those of you who do not particularly like coconut, avocado oil is an excellent substitute.

Fish: Fish provides a good source of omega-3 fatty acids, which are essential to heart health. Take care of your heart and it will take care of you. Favor wild-caught fish, as farmed fish are often not fed their natural diet and therefore aren't as nutritious for you.

Animal Protein: Poultry and grass-fed meats are a critical part of the Paleo Diet. Animal protein is what enabled our ancestors to develop into intelligent human beings and what continues to nourish us today. Animal protein will be a staple both during your Paleo Cleanse and after, if you chose to continue a Paleo lifestyle.

Superfoods: These are foods with high antioxidant levels and nutritional contents, such as acai berries, goji berries, and cacao powder. They are called superfoods for a reason!

All You Can Eat

Vegetables: Suggested vegetable choices for unlimited consumption are listed on the *All You Can Eat Vegetable Buffet* in each week's *Grocery List*.

Paleo in Moderation

Fresh Fruits (high sugar content): While fruits are recommended in virtually unlimited proportions on the Paleo Diet, we recommend restricting the consumption of fruits with high sugar contents during your Paleo Cleanse. This will enable the body to stabilize blood sugar levels and will assist with natural weight loss. During your Paleo Cleanse, minimize your intake of apricots, bananas, grapes, kiwis, melon, and papaya.

Starchy Vegetables: Almost all vegetables are considered Paleo-friendly and therefore are staples on the Paleo Diet. That said, we recommend limiting those vegetables that are high in starch content during your Cleanse. This will also assist in normalizing your blood sugar levels and help you shed any unwanted pounds. Starchy vegetables include yams, sweet potatoes, and some squash varieties.

Grass-fed and Natural Meats (high fat content): While grass-fed and natural meats are a staple of the Paleo Diet, we recommend restricting those with high fat content during your Paleo Cleanse. This will increase your chance for weight loss and help reduce your body fat percentage if you wish to see a noticeable physical change. Post-Cleanse you can be less concerned with fats in grass-fed meats (we'll explain more about this in Chapter 17).

Ghee: Ghee is clarified butter and is very common in Indian cooking. While ghee is a form of dairy, it has become an accepted form of cooking oil on the Paleo Diet, at least according to the more modern schools of Paleo. We recommend restricting your amount of ghee intake during your Cleanse due to its high fat content.

Paleo Flours: Paleo flours are a great substitute to use when baking and cooking. Paleo flours include almond flour, arrowroot flour, coconut flour, and tapioca flour. While on the Paleo Cleanse, we recommend consuming these flours in limited quantities because they are generally high in fat and starch.

Natural Fats: Natural fats found in avocados and nuts are nutrient packed. However, if losing weight and decreasing body fat is a major driver for your Paleo Cleanse journey, we recommend restricting your daily intake of these foods.

Natural Sweeteners: Sweeteners such as coconut palm sugar and honey are great replacements for traditional refined sugar. That said, consuming too much of these substitutes can increase your insulin levels and cause weight gain. We recommend restricting your intake of these sweeteners during your Paleo Cleanse.

Foods to Avoid at All Costs

Dairy: Yogurt, cheese, ice cream, milk. Dairy affects insulin, the skin, and mucous membranes. While some people can tolerate lactose (are lactase persistent), this doesn't change the fact that milk's purpose is to make baby cows grow up quickly. Leave it to the cows. (Note: Some schools of Paleo approve the consumption of grass-fed dairy. We'll discuss this toward the end of the book, but for your Cleanse, dairy should remain off-limits.)

Gluten: Protein found in wheat, barley, rye, beer. Gluten literally means "glue" in Latin. Why would you glue together your gut?

GMOs: GMO stands for Genetically Modified Organism. Need we say more?

Grain: Corn, rice, pasta, bread, cereal, oats. Ever put a loaf of bread in your mouth and sucked on it? It breaks down into pure sugar.

Hormone-Induced Meats: Artificially fattened animals aren't healthy and neither will you be if you consume them.

Industrial Foods: TV dinners, fast foods, hydrogenated foods. Foods that don't go bad in normal timeframes should raise a red flag.

Legumes: Beans, peanuts, lentils, chickpeas, and soybeans cannot be digested properly by the body. Stick to foods your body can absorb nutrients from, and you will avoid digestive complications.

Soda: Pop, fizzy drinks. Whatever you want to call it, it's a big, sugar-overloaded no-no.

Refined Sugar: Cane sugar, refined sugar, syrup, candy. Your cells can only cope with so much insulin before diabetes kicks in.

Vegetable and Seed Oils: Canola oil, sunflower seed oil, corn oil, soybean oil. If it can fuel your car, it shouldn't fuel you.

The Flintstone Test

Don't see a food on these lists and want to know if it's Paleo? Think back to the *Flintstone Test* that we introduced in Chapter 1. *The Flintstone Test* is simple—ask yourself the question: *would a caveman eat it?* You can also ask yourself: *Did the main ingredients exist in the Paleolithic Era?* If you answer no to either of these questions, you should probably stay away from eating it.

CHAPTER 9

Perform a Pantry Purification

A pantry purification is a necessary step in starting your Cleanse, primarily because it will reduce the chances of giving in to cravings. Since cravings can occur anywhere, you'll need to clean out more than just your pantry—any place where you keep food should be cleared. This includes your fridge, pantry, and desk drawers, just to name a few. Clearing everything out will do you three favors: reduce temptation, symbolize your commitment, and provide you with a fresh start.

You're going to need a large trash bag, maybe two! Use the list and checklist on the following page to make sure you don't miss any common items or storage locations.

The following are a few things you'll want to get rid of (for a complete list of Paleo-unfriendly foods, refer back to the *Foods to Avoid at All Costs* section in Chapter 8):

Foods to Throw Out

- Anything with preservatives
- Bread
- Candy
- Cheese
- Crackers
- Creamer
- Dairy
- Flours
- Frozen TV dinners
- Margarine
- Pastries
- Potato chips
- Pretzels
- Soda
- Sugar
- Vegetable oils

Purification Checklist

Pantry	Fridge	Desk Drawer	Gym Bag	Car	Everywhere Else
❏	❏	❏	❏	❏	❏

CHAPTER 10

Stock Up on Paleo Cleanse Foods

At this point, any Paleo-unfriendly foods you might have been hoarding should be on their merry way to the dumpster. No doubt your cupboards and fridge are looking a little empty. Now it's time to refill them with Paleo-friendly foods!

The following is a list of *Paleo Cleanse Essentials* that you should always have on hand. You'll need them during your Cleanse. This is not meant to be a replacement for your weekly *Grocery List*; it is meant as a list of go-to items. Note that proteins, fruits and vegetables for meals have been left out of the *Paleo Cleanse Essentials* list as they will be included in your weekly *Grocery List*.

Paleo Cleanse Essentials List			
Snacks	Oils	Spices	Other
• Almond butter • Dried fruit • Fresh fruit • Jerky • Nuts • Vegetables	• Avocado oil • Coconut oil • Olive oil	• Black pepper • Chili powder • Cumin • Garlic powder • Paprika • Salt	• Almond milk • Cacao powder • Coconut milk • Coconut aminos • Coffee • Tea

We recommend taking the *Paleo Cleanse Essentials* and the Week One *Grocery List* to your local farmer's market, health shop, or grocery store to stock up for the beginning of your Cleanse. Don't be intimidated by shopping Paleo. Like anything, it'll take some time to adjust to. By the end of the Paleo Cleanse you'll be a Paleo food aficionado!

CHAPTER 11

30 Days of Success

We want to make sure that your Paleo Cleanse is successful. The first step to success is commitment. The techniques below will help to get you there.

Commit to a Month

When it comes to anything new, the trick to making it stick is to make it a habit. If you can commit to a month, which is really not that long, you will find success with the Paleo Cleanse.

It's a well-supported fact that someone who commits to something for 21 consecutive days will be far more likely to continue the habit after that date. We know what you're thinking—then why is the Paleo Cleanse 30 days? We think a month is a good length: it Beats the 21-day milestone, and 30 days is a very scalable and achievable number that is easy to track on a calendar. There's no doubt that you can do it for 30 days. We did!

Thirty days is just long enough to witness yourself feeling better, sleeping better, waking up naturally, and not suffering from blood sugar crashes and mood swings. You will begin to feel alert and productive, and exercising will become easier as you have more energy and improved athletic endurance.

It may seem more difficult to quit grains, sugar, dairy, and legumes cold turkey, but that's actually the easier way to begin. After just a few days your cravings for these foods will disappear, and keeping up the trend for the full four weeks will become a lot easier.

It's just a month of your life. Give it a fair shot. Trust us, it will be well worth it; we know from our own experience.

Find a Cleanse Partner

A *Cleanse Partner* is someone with whom you can embark on your Paleo Cleanse journey and share your results. If you can't find a *Cleanse Partner*, see if you can find an *Accountability Buddy*—someone who is willing to support you throughout your Cleanse and hold you accountable.

Having a *Cleanse Partner* or an *Accountability Buddy* is a well-supported method for reaching any goal, and we know from experience that doing something like the Paleo Cleanse with another individual will increase your chances of success dramatically. Even if you don't have a *Cleanse Partner*, you may well find a coworker, friend, or family member who is willing to help create snacks or join you on a cook-up night to keep you company.

Because we worked together daily, we found it was easiest to collaborate on work lunches and snacks. It made it more manageable— we each had less to bring and less to worry about—and we knew we had to bring what we were assigned to, or we would only have half a meal.

A few things that you can do when completing the Paleo Cleanse with someone else include arranging for each of you to make one of the two daily snacks per week or splitting up ingredients for meals (if you work together one of you could bring the protein for lunch and the other could bring the fruits or vegetables). Both of these ideas will cut down on the amount of time you spend shopping for and preparing the food.

Another benefit of sharing the Paleo Cleanse experience with someone else is that they place an unspoken, invisible layer of accountability on you, which you yourself cannot impose. Accountability through pressure is a wonderful thing! Put simply, you'll feel more obligated to stay on track. You can also share your experiences with each other, celebrate your achievements, and encourage each other to stay strong throughout the Cleanse.

Learn to Fight Cravings

Cravings will be natural during your first week or so of the Paleo Cleanse. It's only normal. We got them and at some point you most likely will as well. To make your life easier, here are a few tricks you can try if you start to experience cravings.

First, try not to eat any Paleo-unfriendly foods once you begin your Paleo Cleanse. We know this is easier said than done, but your cravings will go away more quickly in the long run if you don't eat the foods that you are craving now. You've got willpower, so make sure you use it. Usually, after Week One of the Paleo Cleanse your cravings will begin to disappear.

Second, make sure you keep yourself nourished and hydrated. If you stay hydrated and eat the natural, balanced meals that we suggest in the weekly *Meal Plans*, you will find yourself less hungry, with reduced cravings.

Third, there are some great options that you can use as Paleo substitutes if your cravings persist:

- If you're craving sweets, try having a little honey with dried apple, or dates.
- If you're craving soda, try sparkling water or sparkling water with fresh fruit added.
- If you're craving dairy, try coconut milk or almond milk.

- If you're craving potatoes or potato chips, try homemade sweet potato fries, sweet potato chips, or beet chips prepared in coconut oil.

Designate a Grocery Day

Make your life easy, especially during the workweek. One easy way to alleviate Paleo Cleanse prep time is to designate a grocery shopping day. That's why we prepared an easy-to-use weekly *Grocery List* for you. Decide which options on the weekly *Meal Plans* you are going to make, take the list to the store with you, and buy everything at once. This includes all your fresh snack choices, like fruit, eggs, and meat to make the jerky. For dry snacks, such as nuts and dates, we recommend purchasing in bulk, so that these items last at least a month; doing this will also help you save money. We also suggest having dry snacks on hand for emergency nibbling as needed; we'll cover more about this in Chapter 12.

With everything you need for the week, there'll be no excuse to cheat!

Set Cooking Days

Everyone is so busy nowadays that it's hard to make time to do the necessary things in life—like eating well to keep your body healthy. We understand and we've been there. As a tip, we recommend that you set aside a night or two each week for preparing your meals for the week, or at least the next few days. We typically prepare most items for the workweek each Sunday. (We also use Sunday as our grocery-shopping day.)

If you dedicate one day at the beginning of the week and one in the middle for preparing your food for the next few days, you'll be more likely to achieve success on your Paleo Cleanse journey. Eating Paleo doesn't need to be challenging or time consuming; having set cooking days to prepare your meals for the week will help you stay committed and on track.

Learning How to Bake and Cook Paleo-Style

Paleo baking and cooking can be quite the experience if you haven't done either before. We know because we lived it during our Cleanse. First, we had to learn to work with new materials, like coconut oil, arrowroot flour, and flaxseed. Let's just say we did end up throwing a few things out and starting over! We found several Paleo recipes that sounded amazing, but when we looked at the ingredients and the steps involved with making them, we felt overwhelmed. We finally managed to get a handle on things about halfway through our month-long commitment, but that was because we decided to ignore what others were doing and make our own recipes up.

Easy and fast recipes is one area that we have focused on for this Cleanse because we know how difficult it can be to prepare Paleo recipes, especially when you're just getting started. We've created recipes both for during and after the Cleanse that are simple to make and absolutely delicious. You'll be able to purchase the ingredients for these recipes at your local grocery store. You can cook these recipes in a matter of minutes when you get home from work, and you will not be intimidated as there is neither fancy cooking lingo nor overly exotic ingredients. To top it off, we're going to provide you with customizable weekly *Meal Plans* and handy *Grocery Lists* to make your planning and shopping a breeze.

Track Your Progress

Mark the Calendar: Another tool for success that we encourage you to use is a simple calendar to mark off your days. It's always gratifying to see your accomplishments, and with this calendar, you'll be able to see your progress every day during your Cleanse. Simply mark off each day as you complete it. If you happen to be doing your Cleanse on a month with 31 days and want to go the extra step, by all means, take credit for that extra day!

Month:				Year:		
Day 1 ❑	Day 2 ❑	Day 3 ❑	Day 4 ❑	Day 5 ❑	Day 6 ❑	Day 7 ❑
Day 8 ❑	Day 9 ❑	Day 10 ❑	Day 11 ❑	Day 12 ❑	Day 13 ❑	Day 14 ❑
Day 15 ❑	Day 16 ❑	Day 17 ❑	Day 18 ❑	Day 19 ❑	Day 20 ❑	Day 21 ❑
Day 22 ❑	Day 23 ❑	Day 24 ❑	Day 25 ❑	Day 26 ❑	Day 27 ❑	Day 28 ❑
Day 29 ❑	Day 30 ❑	Day 31 ❑				

Keep Your Worksheets Handy: Before beginning Week One of the Paleo Cleanse, make sure that you have filled in the pre-Cleanse worksheets we provided in Chapter 5. This will be essential for when you look back at the end of the full four weeks to see how you've changed. It's important that you filled in those answers honestly based on how you feel on your current diet. Think about it this way: You're the only one who needs to see those sheets, so feel confident enough to be honest with yourself. Once the four weeks of the Cleanse are under your belt and you revisit those worksheets you will have a clear idea of what the Cleanse did for you personally.

Keep a Journal: This journey is all about you. Everyone's body reacts slightly differently and at it's own pace. The changes we covered in Chapters 3 and 4 are the most common benefits experienced. That said, your Cleanse might bring about a different outcome and you may notice other improvements that are worth noting and sharing.

It's interesting to journal about your day-to-day experience on the Cleanse, or to take a few notes on your smartphone or in a notepad. You can jot down when cravings kick in, when they vanish, what you notice after eating pure Paleo lunches, and what your energy levels are telling you about the foods you are eating. Also, if you do happen to cheat or accidentally eat a food you didn't know wasn't Paleo, pay close attention to how your body reacts and how it makes you feel. Keep those notes to reflect upon as you go (and to look back at smiling) once you've completed the full four weeks.

Let's Do This!

You've learned about the Paleo Diet. You know how the Paleo Cleanse originated, why it is successful, and how it works. You just prepared yourself for the Paleo Cleanse. Now it's time to jump straight into Week One. Use the tools we've provided in this book and on ThePaleoPact. com to ensure your continued success. It's time to Paleo Cleanse!

PART 3

THE 30-DAY PALEO CLEANSE

CHAPTER 12

Paleo Cleanse, Week One

Welcome to Week One of the Paleo Cleanse!

Your pantry has been purified and restocked with the *Paleo Cleanse Essentials* and Week One groceries. You've committed to completing the full month of your Paleo Cleanse and you can't wait to feel the positive changes on your body, so you have the right mental attitude as well. You're ready to begin and the fun starts now.

Take it slow and keep it simple. Master the basics and then start experimenting when you feel ready. We will guide you on how to begin experimenting during Week Two, if you wish to do so.

The recipes in Week One's *Meal Plan* are simple and very "clean." There is not a lot of spice, sauce, or fancy concoctions. It's like that for a reason. When we journeyed through Week One we found that simple was the way to go—it just makes the Paleo Cleanse that much more practical and achievable. If you would like to try all the recipes in the Week One *Meal Plan*, that's great, but if you want to be super easy on yourself and stick with repeating just a few of them, that's no problem at all. That way you can cook twice as much at once and save time on your cooking day. Do whatever makes your Paleo Cleanse easiest and most enjoyable for you. And remember, the *All You Can Eat Vegetable Buffet* is essentially a bonus option from which to eat as much as you want, whenever you would like to.

Week One Meal Plan

Since not everyone enjoys the same foods, we designed this *Meal Plan* to be extremely flexible. It's made to be customized, so that you can easily formulate your own Week One *Meal Plan* based on the options listed below and any restrictions you may have personally (such as allergies). As an example, we will provide a list of three breakfast options. You can then pick and choose from that list what you would like to eat each day. It's better for your body to vary your meals to ensure you get a variety of nutrients, but it's okay to eat the same thing each day for the week, if that is preferable to you. The idea is to make this Cleanse as simple as possible to follow so that you have no problem staying committed.

Week One Meal Plan Choices

Monday to Sunday Meal Plan Options		
BREAKFAST	Fruit Salad and Almonds *or* Baked Egg *or* Bacon and Fruit	**BONUS** All You Can Eat Vegetable Buffet!
SNACK	Power Bar *or* Cauliflower Hummus *or* Homemade Jerky *or* Hardboiled Eggs *or* Berries or Fruit *or* Dried Dates *or* Raw Nuts	
LUNCH	Avocado Kale Salad *or* Arugula Protein Salad *or* Lettuce Wraps	
SNACK	Power Bar *or* Cauliflower Hummus *or* Homemade Jerky *or* Hardboiled Eggs *or* Berries or Fruit *or* Dried Dates *or* Raw Nuts	
DINNER	Spaghetti Squash and Sauce *or* Stuffed Butternut *or* Grilled Fish and Vegetables	

Week One Meal Plan Selection

Fill in your personal *Meal Plan* based on the choices above:

PERSONAL MEAL PLAN SELECTION					
	BREAKFAST	**SNACK**	**LUNCH**	**SNACK**	**DINNER**
MONDAY					
TUESDAY					
WEDNESDAY					
THURSDAY					
FRIDAY					

	BREAKFAST	SNACK	LUNCH	SNACK	DINNER
SATURDAY					
SUNDAY					

Week One Grocery List

The below food items share the following in common: all fruits and vegetables should ideally be organic, all meats should preferably be nitrate-free and grass-fed, all poultry and eggs should be free-range, all fish should be wild-caught, olive oil should be extra-virgin, and salt should be non-iodized, if possible (refer back to Chapter 8 if you have any questions about these suggestions).

Breakfast

Option 1: Fruit Salad and Almonds

- apple
- orange or grapefruit
- berries (raspberries, blackberries, and/or blueberries)
- almonds

Option 2: Baked Egg

- coconut oil
- eggs
- black pepper (optional)

Option 3: Bacon and Fruit

- bacon
- apple or orange

Lunch

Option 1: Avocado Kale Salad

- mature or baby kale
- cucumber
- sliced raw almonds
- avocado
- olive oil
- orange
- balsamic vinegar

Option 2: Arugula Protein Salad

- arugula
- olive oil
- orange
- sundried tomatoes
- coconut oil
- chicken breasts
- garlic
- dried oregano
- balsamic vinegar

Option 3: Lettuce Wraps

- coconut oil
- ground beef
- green peppers
- onions
- carrots
- tahini
- lettuce cups
- avocado

Dinner

Option 1: Spaghetti Squash and Sauce

- spaghetti squash
- coconut oil
- yellow onion
- carrot
- tomatoes
- garlic
- black pepper
- Italian seasoning
- salt

Option 2: Stuffed Butternut

- butternut squash
- coconut oil
- ground lamb
- garlic
- tomatoes
- sundried tomatoes
- fresh basil

Option 3: Grilled Fish and Vegetables

- yams
- asparagus
- coconut oil
- fish fillet (halibut, tilapia, trout, or swordfish)
- garlic
- sundried tomatoes
- button mushrooms
- paprika
- lemon

Snacks

Option 1: Power Bars

- walnuts
- raisins
- dried apples
- cinnamon powder
- egg white protein powder

Option 2: Cauliflower Hummus

- cauliflower
- cumin powder
- coconut oil
- garlic (fresh or powdered)
- tahini
- lemons
- olive oil
- carrots

Option 3: Homemade Jerky

- frozen beef roast
- balsamic vinegar
- salt

Option 4: Hardboiled Eggs

- eggs
- coconut oil
- black pepper
- salt

Option 5: Berries or Fruit

- berries (blueberries, blackberries, strawberries, and/or raspberries)
- apple, orange, grapefruit, peach, and/or pear

Option 6: Dried Dates

- dried Medjool dates

Option 7: Raw Nuts

- nuts (almonds, walnuts, cashews, or macadamias)

Option 8: All You Can Eat Vegetable Buffet

- broccoli
- cauliflower
- asparagus
- peppers
- carrots
- cucumber
- eggplant
- celery
- Brussels sprouts

Drink Options

- water
- unsweetened tea
- unsweetened coffee without creamer
- coconut water

If you are not sure of the best place to find any of the above items, refer to the *Purchasing Directory* on page 285.

Week One Recipes

Each of the recipes below makes a single serving, with the exception of the Power Bars, Hummus, and Jerky, which will provide you with four to five servings. If you are preparing your Week One meals in advance, simply multiply the quantity in the below recipes by the number of times you plan to enjoy each recipe during the week.

Breakfast

Fruit Salad and Almonds

Fruit eaten together with nuts ensures constant blood sugar stabilization. Nuts are slower to digest and will help sustain you for longer.

INGREDIENTS

1 apple, chopped into bite-size pieces

1 citrus fruit, sliced into bite-size segments

¼ cup berries

¼ cup almonds

SUPPLIES

measuring cups

sharp knife

breakfast bowl

Place the apple, citrus, and berries in a breakfast bowl.

Stir to mix, then top with almonds and serve.

Baked Egg

Very high in protein and vitamins, eggs provide an excellent source of nourishment to start your day. The yolk is home to fat-soluble vitamins, essential fatty acids, calcium, iron, zinc, phosphorus, and B vitamins.

INGREDIENTS

½ teaspoon coconut oil

1 egg

black pepper (optional)

SUPPLIES

measuring spoon

small ramekin

oven mitts

Preheat the oven to 450°F.

Grease a small ramekin with the coconut oil.

Crack the egg into the ramekin.

Place the container in the oven and bake for 8 to 10 minutes for a marginally soft yolk, or 10 to 12 minutes for a hard yolk.

Remove from the oven, sprinkle with black pepper (if desired), and serve hot.

Bacon and Fruit

Bacon is a great source of B vitamins, zinc, magnesium, and omega-3 fatty acids. Plus, it's delicious! Paired with fruits that are high in fiber, the bacon is more easily digested by the body, helping to mitigate the cholesterol concern.

INGREDIENTS

2 slices bacon

1 apple or orange

SUPPLIES

aluminum foil

baking tray

Preheat the oven to 425°F.

Place the bacon strips on a foil-lined baking sheet and place in the oven for 8 to 10 minutes for cooked bacon, or 10 to 12 minutes for crispy bacon.

Remove from the oven and serve together with your choice of fruit.

Lunch

Avocado Kale Salad

Rich in natural fats and very refreshing, this salad combines avocado with kale, which is claimed to be one of the world's healthiest foods. Kale boasts very high quantities of vitamins A, C, and K, along with various minerals and antioxidants.

INGREDIENTS

2 cups kale

¼ large cucumber, sliced

2 tablespoons raw almonds, sliced

½ avocado, sliced

2 tablespoons olive oil

2 tablespoons freshly squeezed orange juice

2 tablespoons balsamic vinegar

SUPPLIES

measuring cups and spoons

sharp knife

salad bowl

shaker

In a salad bowl, toss the kale, cucumber, and almonds before placing the avocado on the bed of greens.

In a shaker, add the equal parts olive oil, orange juice, and balsamic vinegar and mix or shake until well combined.

Pour the dressing mixture over the salad and serve chilled or at room temperature.

Arugula Protein Salad

Combining protein, natural fats, and fresh greens, this
refreshing salad provides a balanced and delicious meal.

INGREDIENTS

2 cups arugula

1 tablespoon olive oil

1 orange, sliced

⅓ cup sundried tomatoes

1 tablespoon coconut oil

¼ pound chicken breasts, sliced thinly

1 teaspoon garlic, chopped finely

½ teaspoon dried oregano

1 teaspoon balsamic vinegar

SUPPLIES

measuring cups and spoons

sharp knife

medium bowl

medium sauté pan

In a medium bowl, toss the arugula with the olive oil.

Add the orange and sundried tomatoes.

In a medium sauté pan, melt the coconut oil over medium heat.

Add the chicken breast strips, garlic, and oregano and cook over medium
heat for 12 to 15 minutes, until the chicken is well-done.

Once cooked, place the chicken strips on the bed of greens and drizzle
with balsamic vinegar.

Serve while the chicken is hot.

Lettuce Wraps

Lettuce is a great wheat-free wrap alternative. Filled with a protein-rich beef and vegetable combination, this wrap is not only delicious and satisfying, but requires very little prep time.

INGREDIENTS

1 tablespoon coconut oil

¼ pound ground beef

½ cup green peppers, sliced thinly

¼ cup onions, chopped finely

¼ cup carrots, diced

1 teaspoon tahini

3 lettuce leaves

½ avocado, sliced

SUPPLIES

measuring cups and spoons

sharp knife

medium sauté pan

dinner plate

In a medium sauté pan, melt the coconut oil over medium heat.

Add the beef, peppers, onions, carrots, and tahini and cook over medium-high heat for about 10 minutes, stirring occasionally.

Place the lettuce leaves on a dinner plate.

Scoop the beef mixture into the lettuce leaves and top with avocado.

Serve while the beef is hot.

Dinner

Spaghetti Squash and Sauce

A solution to any Italian dinner cravings, this recipe is very
simple to make and provides a quick yet balanced hot meal.

INGREDIENTS

1 cup spaghetti squash, seeded

2 tablespoons coconut oil

1 yellow onion, chopped finely

1 large carrot, sliced thinly

32 ounces finely chopped tomatoes

3 cloves garlic, chopped finely or crushed

1 tablespoon black pepper

2 tablespoons Italian seasoning

1 teaspoon salt (optional)

SUPPLIES

measuring spoons

sharp knife

large pot

medium sauté pan

Bring water to a boil in a large pot.

Place the spaghetti squash in the pot; boil for about 25 minutes, until soft.

Remove the spaghetti squash from the water and allow to cool.

In a medium sauté pan, melt the coconut oil over medium heat.

Add the onion and carrot and cook over medium-high heat until the
onion starts to brown.

Reduce the heat to medium and add the tomatoes, garlic, pepper, Italian
seasoning, and salt.

Cover the pan and let simmer for 15 to 20 minutes.

Scoop the soft spaghetti squash into a serving bowl.

Pour the sauce mixture over the spaghetti squash and serve hot.

Stuffed Butternut

South African–style lamb-stuffed butternut squash is one of our favorite dishes to whip up when time is of the essence. The butternut acts as a starch alternative and pairs perfectly with the tender lamb flavors.

INGREDIENTS

½ (2 pound) butternut squash, seeded

1 tablespoon coconut oil

¼ pound ground lamb

1 garlic clove, chopped finely

¼ cup fresh tomatoes, diced

1 tablespoon sundried tomatoes, sliced thinly

1 tablespoon fresh basil, chopped

SUPPLIES

measuring cup and spoon

sharp knife

large pot

medium sauté pan

Bring water to a boil in a large pot.

Place the butternut squash in the pot and boil for about 15 to 20 minutes, until tender.

In a medium sauté pan, melt the coconut oil over medium heat.

Add the lamb and cook for about 5 minutes, tossing intermittently.

Add the garlic, fresh tomatoes, and sundried tomatoes and cook for another 5 minutes, stirring occasionally.

Toss the basil on the lamb mixture and let simmer for another minute.

Place the butternut on a plate, open side up.

Scoop the lamb mixture into the butternut half and enjoy hot.

Grilled Fish and Vegetables

Fish provides an excellent source of Omega-3 fatty acids, calcium, phosphorus, and minerals. It's brain food at its best and, paired with a colorful assortment of vegetables, makes a very healthy meal.

INGREDIENTS

¼ cup thinly sliced yams

¼ pound asparagus, ends clipped

1 tablespoon coconut oil

1 fish fillet (halibut, tilapia, trout, or swordfish)

1 teaspoon crushed garlic

1 tablespoon sundried tomatoes, sliced thinly

¼ cup button mushrooms, sliced thinly

1 teaspoon paprika (optional)

1 lemon

SUPPLIES

measuring cups

sharp knife

large pot

medium sauté pan

Bring water to a boil in a large pot.

Place the yams and asparagus spears into the pot and boil for about 10 to 15 minutes.

In a medium sauté pan, melt the coconut oil over medium heat.

Place the fish fillet in the pan and cook the first side for about 4 minutes.

Flip the fillet, add the garlic, sundried tomatoes, and button mushrooms and cook for another 5 to10 minutes, depending on thickness.

Once the fish is well-done, place on a plate and sprinkle with paprika as desired.

Place the yams and asparagus alongside the fish and squeeze a lemon over the entire dish.

Serve while hot.

Snacks

Power Bars

"Power" is a word that has been associated with the body for decades. In South Africa, the indigenous people use the term to describe the energy derived from food sources. They have it right! We need to eat nutrients in order to power our bodies and minds, not the other way around.

INGREDIENTS

1¼ cup walnuts

1 cup raisins

½ cup dried apples

½ teaspoon cinnamon powder

⅓ cup egg white protein powder

¼ cup water

SUPPLIES

measuring cups

food processor

large glass dish

Place the walnuts in a food processor and pulse for about 20 seconds, or until granular.

Add the raisins, apples, cinnamon powder, protein powder, and water and pulse for about 45 seconds, or until thoroughly combined.

Scoop out the mixture and press into a square or rectangular dish. An 8x8-inch pan makes 10 to 12 half-inch-thick power bars.

Cut the pressed mixture into your desired serving size and place the dish in the refrigerator to set for about an hour.

Serve immediately or keep refrigerated and snack on these bars throughout the week.

Cauliflower Hummus

Thought you'd have to give up hummus on the Paleo Diet?
Think again! This recipe offers a delicious Paleo-friendly
alternative to traditional legume-based hummus.

INGREDIENTS

1 head of cauliflower, cored and cut into quarter-size florets

2 tablespoons cumin powder

1½ tablespoons coconut oil, melted

4 cloves garlic, halved

½ cup tahini

2 lemons, squeezed

¼ cup water

¼ cup olive oil

5 carrots, for dipping

SUPPLIES

measuring cups

sharp knife

large mixing bowl

medium oven-safe dish

food processor

Preheat the oven to 450°F.

In a large mixing bowl, mix the cauliflower florets, cumin, coconut oil, and garlic (you may want to use your hands).

Pour the mixture into a baking dish.

Place in the oven to bake for about 30 minutes, or until the cauliflower turns light golden brown.

Remove from the oven and let cool for about 10 minutes.

Place the cauliflower mixture into your food processor.

Add the tahini, lemon juice, and water and blend until smooth.

Scrape the sides of the processor to ensure the mixture is blended thoroughly.

Stream in the olive oil and pulse for about a minute.

Serve warm, or refrigerate and serve chilled within four days.

Use carrots for dipping.

TIP: For a less garlicky version, replace the fresh garlic with garlic powder. This is recommended if you plan to enjoy the hummus over a couple of days.

Homemade Jerky

You probably thought jerky would be a Paleo no-brainer. Think again! Most store-bought jerky has copious amounts of wheat and soy. Don't worry; we've got you covered with this easy recipe.

INGREDIENTS

1 (4- to 5-pound) frozen beef roast

1 (8- to 10-ounce) bottle balsamic vinegar

1 teaspoon salt

SUPPLIES

measuring spoon

sharp knife

marinade bowl

aluminum foil

baking sheet

Place the frozen roast out to defrost until the outside rim of the roast is soft but the center is still slightly frozen.

Slice the roast into strips that are about ⅛-inch thick, then place the strips in a bowl.

Pour enough balsamic vinegar into the bowl to almost cover the beef strips.

Sprinkle with salt and stir until the marinade coats all the beef.

Allow the mixture to sit and marinate for at least two hours (overnight in the refrigerator is better if time allows).

Preheat the oven to 190°F.

Place the beef strips onto a foil-lined baking sheet.

Place in the oven to bake and flip about every 30 minutes.

To test if the jerky is done, fold a piece in half and look for white threads. If you see them the jerky is cooked.

Once done, remove the jerky from the oven and allow to cool before serving, or refrigerate and enjoy within 5 days.

TIP: Make sure you cut the jerky thin enough; otherwise, you'll get little, not so tasty steaks. Also, having the meat slightly frozen will make it easier to cut. Use a serrated knife and keep hot water running to run your hands under—they will get cold!

Hardboiled Eggs

Eggs provide a fantastic source of protein, are easy to prepare in advance, and, when you eat the yolk, provide your body with an abundance of vitamins and nutrients. Snack happily and don't worry about the cholesterol: There is actually no clear evidence to show that eggs have any impact on cardiovascular disease.

INGREDIENTS

1 egg

1 teaspoon coconut oil

½ teaspoon black pepper

½ teaspoon salt

SUPPLIES

measuring spoons

small pot

small sauté pan

Bring water to a boil in a small pot.

Place the egg in the boiling water and cook for about 12 minutes.

Remove the egg from the pot and allow to cool for about 5 minutes.

In small sauté pan, melt the coconut oil over medium heat.

Pour the melted coconut oil into a small bowl and then mix in the black pepper and salt.

Peel the eggshell and dip the egg in the coconut, pepper, and salt mixture.
Place in the refrigerator and enjoy within four days.

Berries or Fruit

Berries or a piece of fruit make a great, quick snack and an excellent
substitute for any Week One sugar cravings you might experience.

While there is no specific recipe for this snack option, enjoy
either ¼ cup of berries (blueberries, blackberries, strawberries, and/
or raspberries) or a piece of fruit (an apple, orange, grapefruit, peach,
or pear). These fruits were specifically chosen because they have lower
fructose levels. You don't see bananas, melons, and grapes on this
list because those fruits are very high in natural sugar and should
be avoided during the Paleo Cleanse. Post-Cleanse, we recommend
consuming those sugary fruits in moderation.

Dried Dates

Dates are very nutritious and naturally sweet, making them a
worthwhile snack to have on hand, especially during Week One. Dates
are high in fiber, iron, vitamin A, and vitamin K, helping the body
with digestion and providing it with the nutrients necessary to fight
infection. We recommend a portion size of four to six naturally dried
and pitted Medjool dates as a snack option during the Paleo Cleanse.

Raw Nuts

Nuts serve as a natural fat and provide an excellent source of omega-3,
antioxidants, and minerals. Not all nuts are considered Paleo, such as
peanuts, which are not actually a nut and fall into the legume family.
Stick to almonds, walnuts, cashews, or macadamia nuts that are raw,
unsalted, and unsweetened (that's right—no cheating with caramelized
or chocolate-covered nuts!) The recommended serving size of nuts as a
snack option during the Paleo Cleanse is ¼ cup. Keep your nut intake

per day moderate if possible; nuts in excess of ¼ cup a day have been shown to prevent weight loss.

All You Can Eat Vegetable Buffet

Vegetables are extremely healthy for you and provide many necessary nutrients. That's why we've included a buffet category of vegetables that can be enjoyed in any quantity. For a full list of vegetables included in this buffet, refer to the *Grocery List*.

Beverages

Enjoy water, unsweetened tea, coffee without creamer, and coconut water, as you please.

Week One: Overcoming Obstacles

We know how it is: Life gets busy, things come up, and suddenly you have no time to cook. That's when you find yourself at the nearest take-out restaurant for dinner and the downward spiral begins. It's okay—we've been there—and sometimes when things get hectic we still (to this day) resort to takeout sushi. But just for this month, take life by the reins and show it that no matter what it throws at you, you can still follow the Paleo Cleanse.

The best way to ensure nothing disrupts your schedule is to prepare in advance. That way, if you run into a time lock or have to work late and can't get your cooking in, it's no big deal—you will have done it already.

Always Eat Breakfast

You know that saying "Breakfast is the most important meal of the day"? Well, it's not something that's actually agreed upon by all nutritionists. Nonetheless, it's a notion that we believe to be very important, particularly during the Paleo Cleanse. Why? Eating breakfast kick-starts your metabolism, stabilizes your blood sugar, and prevents cheating. The thing is, this concept is lost on the traditional Western Diet: Consuming cereal with skim milk in the morning or toast with jelly is not going to do your body the good it needs, nor is it providing sustenance for your day. What it's really providing is a guaranteed blood sugar crash in just a few short hours.

The breakfasts included in the Paleo Cleanse are protein- and fiber-rich, low in sugar, and free of starch, so your body can get to work quickly on digesting your breakfast and be ready to digest your next meal or snack. Your blood sugar level normalizes right from the get-go (something that isn't the case with carbohydrate- and sugar-based breakfasts) and you aren't hungry before the day begins, which eliminates the chance of bad snacking. Eating your breakfast is like starting your day off on the right foot.

Drink Plenty of Water

More than 60 percent of the human body is composed of water. You are constantly losing fluid through sweat, evaporation, etc., and you need to ensure you replace it. The rule of drinking "eight glasses a day" for optimal health is actually debatable, and you will likely find that on the Paleo Diet, you will be less thirsty (Paleo-friendly foods contain natural water and have less sugar and salt). That being said, you still need to provide your body with the water it needs to function. Water is necessary for digestion, circulation, nutrient transportation, saliva creation, and even body temperature regulation. Water is also a great way to aid your body in flushing out toxins—something that is particularly beneficial during Week One of the Paleo Cleanse.

Throw Away Any Temptations

We know you took care of your pantry already, but think beyond that to anything that may set your mind down the road of guilty pleasures. For example, we both have a "Million Dollar Bar" chocolate on our desks. It took us a while to get past the fact that it was of course edible (and is probably delicious) and look at it simply as a token of financial freedom. Candy-stocked desk bowls, bubble gum, flavored ChapStick, scented candles, and sugary lotions can sometimes be enough to trigger a craving. Get rid of it all (or at least what you're willing to in the beginning). Make the Cleanse as easy as you can by avoiding all possible triggers.

Fight Snack Attacks

You'll notice that there are three options for each meal category (breakfast, lunch, and dinner), as well as several snack options in case you get hungry between meals. The snack options are positioned between breakfast and lunch, and between lunch and dinner. Try to only snack between these times. If you have to snack after dinner, look to the *All You Can Eat Vegetable Buffet*. Remember that to sleep optimally your body needs to have finished digesting your food before it can rest and rejuvenate for the next day; the *All You Can Eat Vegetable Buffet* is the best choice to support this if you have to eat after dinner.

Week One is the week that you are most likely to feel hungry between meals and experience food cravings. This will happen because you still have residual effects in your system caused by the foods from your previous diet. Until your body has processed those foods completely, you can expect to have some cravings (this is common in the case of sugar and carbohydrates). Just go into Week One expecting this to occur and don't get despondent over it. Decide what snacks sound most delicious to you and prepare them in advance (see *Store Snacks in Bulk*, on the following page). Select some options that don't require refrigeration and carry them with you. Don't wait until the point that you are starving because this will be the instance where you are most likely to cheat. It's okay to snack often, especially from the *All You Can Eat Vegetable Buffet* list.

Remember, this is not a starvation cleanse. This *Meal Plan* is built around foods that our bodies can easily digest and which don't include grains, legumes, dairy, or refined sugars. Your body doesn't need to be starved in order to be cleansed. It will realign and rebalance itself with the help of nutritional foods. So we're going to say it: "Eat up!" and don't feel guilty about it for a second.

Store Snacks in Bulk

If you were ever to snoop in our desk drawers, you would find no papers, minimal stationary, a couple of flash drives, and a whole lot of snack food. Seriously, between the two of us, we could feed ourselves for a month on snacks alone; it's our secret to sticking to our Paleo lifestyle.

During your 30-Day Paleo Cleanse we highly recommend that you become snack hoarders like us and curveball any cravings by having a great variety of Paleo Cleanse snacks on hand at all times. Yes, we are suggesting that you carry some snacks in your bag, too—you never know when hunger will kick in.

You may be wondering where such experienced snack hoarders purchase their stash. The truth is, we get most of it from Costco. There you will find giant bags of almonds, walnuts, dates, and other dried fruits—it's like a snack-hoarders heaven. So stock up and have plenty from the *All You Can Eat Vegetable Buffet* in both your work and home refrigerators, and you will be super-prepared for Week One and beyond.

Prevent Allergies

If you have a food allergy, you're probably already used to experimenting because you've been forced into it. If Week One recipes, or any in this book, contain a food that you are allergic or sensitive to, experiment with switching it out for alternate Paleo-friendly foods. Chapter 20 is there to help you; it includes several substitutes for common food allergens.

Join the Paleo Community

There are many great websites, blogs, and social networks dedicated to the Paleo lifestyle. We encourage you to visit them, get ideas, be inspired, and meet other people who, just like you, are committed to health.

Our own website, ThePaleoPact.com, our Facebook page, "The Paleo Pact," and our Twitter page, @ThePaleoPact, are jam-packed with free recipes, Paleo resources, hot topics, and links to great research articles. We keep it light-hearted and interesting in the hope of helping you stay motivated. We encourage you to comment, discuss your challenges, and share your best practices and favorite recipes with the community—it's helpful for everyone and it's so much easier when you're not going through a new adventure alone.

Be Prepared for Questions

Your diet is suddenly completely different and you turn down the mid-morning bagel run and late-night dessert trip. Your friends, family, and coworkers start to wonder what's up. At first they think you're just not feeling well, and when you break the news about the Paleo Cleanse, they say something like, "Oh, isn't that like Atkins? It's that caveman thing right? Isn't it a fad diet?"

That's when you take a deep breath and respond with a calculated answer. Not everyone will agree with you or think it's a good idea, so refrain from being judgmental or condemning Paleo-unfriendly foods. Simply state that you are committed to a 30-Day Cleanse in which you will be eating all-natural foods, eliminating carbohydrates, and reducing your sugar intake. It's hard to argue with that! If you keep your attack against industrial foods rather than grains, legumes, and dairy (things that most people don't like the thought of giving up), then it's so much easier for others to understand and support.

As you progress through the four weeks and possibly beyond, you will no doubt be approached with more questions. To help you with this, we have included a section dedicated to this precise topic in Chapter 19, titled *FAQ and Paleo Answers*.

Always Have Extra Staples On Hand

Nothing makes a cleanse harder than finding yourself hungry and not having anything healthy to eat. Vending machines, coffee shop snacks, and drive-throughs are now off-limits, so plan well and stock your bag with an assortment of options from the Week One snack menu to tide you over between meals, even when you're on the go.

Don't Wait Until You're Hungry

Remember, the Paleo Cleanse is not meant to starve you, so if you need a snack, enjoy one of the snack options. If you need more, indulge in the *All You Can Eat Vegetable Buffet*.

During Week One you will still have a residue of grains, dairy, and legumes in your body and subsequently will likely experience some initial cravings and withdrawals from those foods. This also means that you may experience sugar highs and lows during Week One, but these will subside as those foods pass through your body. A great way to get ahead of the game is to eat before you are starving. You don't have to eat a lot, nor should you eat much unless you are truly hungry, but it does not hurt to munch on a carrot or broccoli crown every now and then, keeping the dreaded sugar surges at bay.

Eating regularly during Week One will keep your metabolism working hard, so the unwanted foods can pass quickly through your body and full-blown Paleo can take over in Week Two. By understanding that it takes time and that Week One is the biggest hurdle, you can be prepared, keep yourself nourished, and stay on track.

Don't Rely On Eating Out

Refraining from eating out during the Cleanse is not easy; we fully admit that. It's especially hard during Week One, when you are still trying to figure out what you can and cannot eat. The solution might not be favorable, but it really is quite simple: Prepare your own food. Restaurants and takeouts may be appealing, but they don't promise the quality and combinations you need for your Paleo Cleanse to be truly successful.

If You Have to Eat Out, Choose Wisely

We know that you may have made prior commitments or that events come up: a birthday party, a business dinner, or a date night. Don't deprive yourself, but be smart about your selection. If at all possible, choose a venue that has lean options, salads, or vegetable sides. Sushi is a good option—you can request the low-carbohydrate, rice-free maki. Grilled fish, grilled chicken, or steak are other good alternatives. Just keep it simple and try to stick to something that is simply meat and vegetables. If you can, ask the server to tell the chef that you're severely allergic to vegetable oils! Kidding aside, if possible, avoid any restaurant oils and butters, steering clear of gravies, batters, and desserts.

Prepare for the Expense

Be prepared to spend more at the grocery store than normal; this expense will decrease as the weeks go by and you figure out what you're doing. We share tip towards the end of this book on places to purchase Paleo foods economically, but it's realistic to expect that regardless of where you shop, your bill is likely to increase a little. It's easy and inexpensive to fill up on bread, pasta, and cereal; it takes larger quantities and more expense to fill up on vegetables and meats. Not to mention that organic, grass-fed, and free-range products are higher priced, but there is a reason for that. When you stare down at your grocery receipt with wide eyes, remember what we talked about in Chapter 3: Your health is worth it and it will cost you a whole lot less in the long run.

Get to Know Your Blood Sugar

Your blood sugar is going to level out as your body is cleansed of excess sugar and starch. As this happens, you will find yourself feeling more balanced, with fewer food-induced mood swings, headaches, and cravings. Pay attention to what your body is telling you and try to snack before you reach a blood sugar low. The sugar crashes will eventually stop as your blood sugar stabilizes. When you reach that point, it's going to feel awesome—just be prepared to feel hungry at odd times and possibly experience withdrawal-like symptoms before you arrive there.

Admit That It's Not That Bad

So you've made it through the first few days and you start to realize this Paleo Cleanse endeavor is really not that bad. You experience a few withdrawal cravings and you're a little hungry, but it's really not the end of the world like you had imagined. Plus, although you're not fully ready to admit it quite yet, you are starting to feel, well, awesome!

Learn to Smile and Laugh It Off

Your friends now call you Flintstone and tease you about hunting down your meals. That's when you simply smile and laugh it off. Better yet, you go along with it. Tell them this Paleo Cleanse meal you're eating is well deserved after the five-mile run it took to conquer your target, followed by the hours of vegetable picking along your return. A mockery embraced is a mockery killed!

Week One Summary

Congratulations! You have officially completed Week One of the Paleo Cleanse. The biggest hurdle is now behind you. Plus, you proved that you could commit to a week of clean eating, so just keep committing to one week at a time.

Before we move on to Week Two, take a moment to review your Week One journey. *Were their certain times of the day that you felt most hungry? Did you experience any cravings or sugar crashes? Were there some recipes that made you feel more satisfied than others?* Your experience on the Paleo Cleanse will be unique, and as you move on to the next three weeks, it pays to know what worked and didn't work for you. Then focus on what did work and be proactive with things that didn't. If you found that you were hungry shortly after breakfast, but ran into a problem finding time to snack before morning meetings, maybe you need to have a few nuts on your way to work. Or if you had a sweet tooth after dinner, maybe you need to have a few fresh berries right after dinner, instead of as an afternoon snack. Now that you've completed a week and have some Paleo Cleanse experience under your belt, all you need to do is rinse and repeat.

You will also be happy to know that Week One is the adjustment phase and that as you proceed to Week Two, your body is likely rid of your pre-Cleanse food buildup and is now being fueled entirely by the healthy Paleo food you are feeding it. With that change comes mood, body, and energy changes, so it's important to note that your experiences in Week Two will likely be very different from Week One. Also vital to note is that you will probably need less food moving forward (unless you increase your exercise), as sugary cravings will subside and Paleo foods are high in protein and will naturally sustain you for longer. You will no doubt also start to sleep better, and with a sounder sleep comes a sharper mind and reduced reliance on food as booster energy. With that in mind, let your body go a little longer sometimes before snacking and take note of how you feel. You don't need to starve yourself—just eat according to the *Meal Plan* and snack on the *All You Can Eat Vegetable Buffet* as often as you like. Constantly listen to your body for what it really needs.

Here's a summary of what you learned in Week One:

- Complete your worksheets from Chapter 5, have a note-taking system in place, and journal about your experience.
- Using the *Meal Plan* options provided, create your own *Meal Plan* for the week.
- Allocate a grocery-shopping day and bring the *Grocery List* with you.
- Stock up on snacks and find an *Accountability Buddy*.
- Stay hydrated, don't skip breakfast, and toss all temptations.
- Join a Paleo community and visit ThePaleoPact.com to stay motivated.
- Try not to eat out, but choose wisely when you do.
- Keep an upbeat attitude and learn to laugh with your critics.

CHAPTER 13

Paleo Cleanse, Week Two

Welcome to Week Two of the Paleo Cleanse! Things are about to get exciting. We're going to go a little off our beaten path from Week One and experiment with what Paleo foods can offer us. You'll find some interesting variations on the foods you enjoyed last week, as well as some creative recipes to play with. Don't worry, though, we're going to keep this simple and short so you can fit it all into your busy schedule.

Keep Your List of Paleo Cleanse Foods Handy

Since you're going to be experimenting with some new recipes this week, it's a good idea to take a look back at the summary of *Cleanse Foods*, *All You Can Eat*, *Paleo in Moderation*, and *Foods to Avoid at All Costs* from Chapter 8. Take some time to reacquaint yourself with these foods; this will help to ensure that as you experiment, you are sticking within the boundaries of your Paleo Cleanse. You may even want to take these lists with you to the grocery store; they will come in handy when reading food labels, which is a necessary component and something we will discuss in more detail later on in this chapter.

Let Go and Have Fun

This week is dedicated to experimenting with food, some of which may be outside of your norm. Commit to letting go this week and trying some new things. Also, don't get upset if an experiment doesn't go the way you plan. We've had our fair share of those incidents! Laugh it off and try again; it may take a time or two before you figure out what works for you.

Week Two Meal Plan

As with Week One, the *Meal Plan* below is customizable. Select what you would like to eat for the week and fill out your Meal Plan Selection chart. You can then carry this around to remind you of exactly what you should be eating and when.

You'll probably notice similar meal choices to last week. Not to worry, they've been adjusted to make them a little more interesting. Our goal is to get you familiar with the basic recipes so that you feel comfortable making variations; that way, you can easily cook with what you have on hand after the Cleanse as well. You may also choose to enjoy some of the recipes from Week One. The extent to which you choose to get creative is entirely up to you.

Week Two Meal Plan Choices

Monday to Sunday Meal Plan Options		
BREAKFAST	Berry Smoothie *or* Omelet Muffins *or* Sausage Patties *or* anything from Week One Breakfasts	**BONUS** All You Can Eat Vegetable Buffet!
SNACK	Blueberry Mango Power Bars *or* Red Pepper Cauliflower Hummus *or* Teriyaki Jerky *or* Berries or Fruit *or* Dried Dates *or* Raw Nuts *or* anything from Week One Snacks	
LUNCH	Lox Salad *or* Roast Beef Wrap-Ups *or* Squash Soup *or* anything from Week One Lunches	
SNACK	Blueberry Mango Power Bars *or* Red Pepper Cauliflower Hummus *or* Teriyaki Jerky *or* Berries or Fruit *or* Dried Dates *or* Raw Nuts *or* anything from Week One Snacks	
DINNER	Burger on a Bed of Arugula *or* Chicken Kebab *or* Grilled Portobello with Pesto *or* anything from Week One Dinners	

Week Two Meal Plan Selection

Fill in your personal *Meal Plan* based on the choices above:

PERSONAL MEAL PLAN SELECTION					
	BREAKFAST	**SNACK**	**LUNCH**	**SNACK**	**DINNER**
MONDAY					
TUESDAY					

	BREAKFAST	SNACK	LUNCH	SNACK	DINNER
WEDNESDAY					
THURSDAY					
FRIDAY					
SATURDAY					
SUNDAY					

Week Two Grocery List

As we stated during Week One, all fruits and vegetables should ideally be organic, all meats should preferably be nitrate-free and grass-fed, all poultry and eggs should be free-range, all fish should be wild-caught, olive oil should be extra-virgin, and salt should be non-iodized, if possible (refer back to Chapter 8 if you have any questions about these suggestions).

Breakfast

Option 1: Berry Smoothie
- banana
- berries (blueberries, blackberries, strawberries, and/or raspberries)
- cinnamon
- coconut milk or almond milk
- egg white protein powder (optional)
- ice

Option 2: Omelet Muffins
- coconut oil
- eggs
- coconut milk
- black pepper (optional)
- salt (optional)
- tomato
- onion

Option 3: Sausage Patties
- honey
- ground pork
- Italian seasoning
- salt (optional)
- coconut oil

Lunch

Option 1: Lox Salad

- arugula
- avocado
- Paleo Caesar Dressing (see page 267)
- lox

Option 2: Roast Beef Wrap-Ups

- avocado
- cherry tomatoes
- cilantro
- red onion
- garlic powder
- paprika
- salt (optional)
- lime
- roast beef

Option 3: Squash Soup

- delicata squash
- orange
- celery
- dried lemongrass/lemongrass spice
- coconut milk

Dinner

Option 1: Burger on a Bed of Arugula

- arugula
- orange
- olive oil
- coconut oil
- ground beef
- dried oregano

Option 2: Chicken Kebab
- coconut aminos
- honey
- garlic
- chicken breasts
- vegetables (your choice from the *All You Can Eat Vegetable Buffet*)

Option 3: Grilled Portobello with Pesto
- portobello mushrooms
- coconut oil
- salt (optional)
- basil
- garlic
- pine nuts
- olive oil
- black pepper (optional)
- salad (your choice of greens)
- cherry tomatoes
- white balsamic vinegar

Snacks

Option 1: Blueberry Mango Power Bars
- walnuts
- dried blueberries
- dried mango
- cinnamon powder
- egg white protein powder (optional)

Option 2: Red Pepper Cauliflower Hummus
- red bell pepper
- cauliflower

- cumin powder
- coconut oil
- garlic (fresh or powdered)
- tahini
- lemons
- olive oil
- carrots

Option 3: Teriyaki Jerky
- frozen beef roast
- balsamic vinegar
- coconut aminos
- salt
- honey

Option 4: Berries or Fruit
- berries (blueberries, blackberries, strawberries, and/or raspberries)
- apple
- orange
- grapefruit
- peach
- pear

Option 5: Dried Dates
- dried Medjool dates
- almond butter (optional)

Option 6: Raw Nuts
- nuts (almonds, walnuts, cashews, or macadamia nuts)

Option 7: All You Can Eat Vegetable Buffet

- broccoli
- cauliflower
- asparagus
- peppers
- carrots
- cucumber
- eggplant
- celery
- Brussels sprouts

Drink Options

- water
- unsweetened tea
- unsweetened coffee without creamer
- coconut water

If you are not sure of the best place to find any of the above items, refer to the *Purchasing Directory* in the back of this book.

Week Two Recipes

Each of the recipes below makes a single serving, with the exception of the Power Bars, Hummus, and Jerky, which will provide you with four to five servings. If you are preparing your Week Two meals in advance, simply multiply the quantity in the below recipes by the number of times you plan to enjoy each recipe during the week.

Breakfast

Berry Smoothie

Bananas and berries offer an excellent dose of natural energy to help get your body up and going in the morning. Not only are these smoothies easy to make, they're also easy to get creative with. Try adding superfoods or natural juice flavors to spice up your mornings.

INGREDIENTS

1 banana

⅓ cup berries

½ teaspoon cinnamon powder

⅓ cup coconut milk or almond milk

⅓ cup egg white protein powder (optional)

5 ice cubes

SUPPLIES

measuring cups

blender

to-go cup

Place the banana, berries, cinnamon, milk, protein powder, and ice in a blender.

Blend until smooth.

Pour into your to-go container and you're ready to walk out the door!

Omelet Muffins

Omelets are a breakfast tradition. These omelet muffins will keep you on track and fueled throughout the morning. They're a great source of protein too!

INGREDIENTS

coconut oil, for greasing

1 egg

1 tablespoon coconut milk

black pepper (optional)

salt (optional)

1 tablespoon chopped tomato

1 tablespoon chopped onion

SUPPLIES

measuring spoons

muffin tin

sharp knife

mixing bowl

whisk

Preheat the oven to 450°F.

Grease two slots of the muffin tin with coconut oil.

Whisk together the egg, milk, black pepper, and salt in a mixing bowl.

Add the tomato and onion to the egg mixture and stir briefly.

Pour the egg mixture into two of the muffin tin slots. Cook for 10 to 12 minutes or until the eggs are thoroughly cooked.

Enjoy warm.

Sausage Patties

Sausage patties are an easy, fast, and smart breakfast choice. They're packed with protein for powering through until your first snack of the day. An added benefit is you can easily make enough to stock up for a few days.

INGREDIENTS

2 tablespoons honey

½ pound ground pork

2 tablespoons Italian seasoning

½ teaspoon salt (optional)

1 tablespoon coconut oil

SUPPLIES

measuring spoons

medium mixing bowl

small plate

medium sauté pan

spatula

Place the honey, ground pork, Italian seasoning, and salt in a mixing bowl and combine thoroughly.

Using your hands, shape the mixture into small (about 2 inches in diameter) patties and place the patties on a plate.

Melt the coconut oil in a sauté pan over medium heat.

Place the patties in the pan and cook for 5 to 8 minutes, until well-done, turning periodically.

Serve warm or refrigerate and reheat if you wish to enjoy them at a later time.

Lunch

Lox Salad

A lox salad is a great way to boost your omega-3 and healthy fat intake. Not only will this fuel you until dinner, but it is also light and satisfying.

INGREDIENTS
1½ cups arugula

½ avocado, sliced

Paleo Caesar Dressing (see page 267)

3 to 4 ounces lox

SUPPLIES
measuring cups

sharp knife

Place the arugula on a plate.

Place the avocado strips on top of the bed of arugula.

Add the dressing and lox to the salad, and toss gently before serving.

Roast Beef Wrap-Ups

Roast beef wrap-ups are one of the easiest lunches possible.
To top it off, you can simply switch the roast beef for turkey or
chicken to change it up a little if you're getting bored. You can even
experiment with adding some vegetables (from the *All You Can Eat
Vegetable Buffet*) to this dish to fill you up more, if needed.

INGREDIENTS

1 avocado

4 cherry tomatoes, quartered

3 sprigs cilantro, chopped

¼ red onion, diced

½ tablespoon garlic powder

½ tablespoon paprika

½ teaspoon salt (optional)

1 lime, squeezed

½ pound roast beef slices

SUPPLIES

measuring spoons

sharp knife

medium mixing bowl

potato masher or fork

Cut the avocado in half and scoop the flesh into the mixing bowl.

Place the cherry tomatoes, cilantro, and red onion into the bowl.

Add garlic powder, paprika, and salt to taste.

Squeeze the juice of one lime over the mixture. Mash with a potato
masher (or fork) until your desired consistency is reached.

Lay out the slices of roast beef, spread the avocado mixture on each
slice, and roll up to enjoy as a wrap.

Squash Soup

This soup is delicious and sure to keep you warm on a cold day.
Served cold, it'll be refreshing on a hot day. It has minimal ingredients
and you can use a Crock-Pot, which always makes things easier!

INGREDIENTS

1½ cups chopped delicata squash

grated zest of ½ orange

½ cup chopped celery

1 teaspoon dried lemongrass/lemongrass spice

1 tablespoon coconut milk

SUPPLIES

measuring cup and spoons

sharp knife

large pot

strainer

slow cooker

Bring water to a boil in a large pot.

Place the squash in the boiling water and cook for 10 to 15 minutes, or
until tender.

Strain the squash and place it in a slow cooker on high, together with all
the other ingredients.

Allow to cook slowly for about 40 minutes to an hour, stirring
occasionally.

Serve hot or refrigerate and enjoy chilled.

Dinner

Burger on a Bed of Arugula

Burgers are a great option when eating Paleo (minus the traditional wheat bun, that is). The best part about burgers is that we all know how to make them. This makes experimenting with them that much easier, and this recipe is a great spin on the traditional burger.

INGREDIENTS

1 cup arugula

1 orange, cut in half

1 teaspoon olive oil

1 tablespoon coconut oil

¼ pound ground beef

1 teaspoon dried oregano

SUPPLIES

measuring spoons

sharp knife

medium sauté pan

Place the arugula on a plate and drizzle with the juice of half an orange and the olive oil.

In a sauté pan, melt the coconut oil over medium heat.

Form the ground beef into a burger patty and place in the pan.

Cook for 2 minutes, then flip and cook to desired preparation.

Sprinkle with oregano and serve warm on the bed of arugula.

Chicken Kebab

This chicken dish is easy to prepare and delicious. With this dish you'll start to experiment with using coconut aminos as a substitute for standard soy sauce. When you master this recipe you'll have a great alternative teriyaki sauce, which you can use for any future dish.

INGREDIENTS

½ cup coconut aminos

¼ cup honey

2 tablespoons garlic, chopped finely

1 pound chicken breast

vegetables, chopped (your choice from the *All You Can Eat Vegetable Buffet*)

SUPPLIES

measuring cups

sharp knife

medium mixing bowl

wooden skewers

grill

Mix the coconut aminos, honey, and diced garlic in a mixing bowl, then set aside.

Cut the chicken breast into bite-size cubes and place in the amino mixture. Stir and let marinate for about 30 minutes.

Using wooden skewers, begin skewering your chicken and vegetables, alternating between the chicken and vegetable pieces.

Grill over medium heat until the chicken is well-done and enjoy hot.

Grilled Portobello with Pesto

Portobellos are a fantastic option to cook with if you decide you want a meat-free meal. They are hearty and packed full of nutrients so they'll fill you up in a good way. The following is an interesting twist on cooking with portobello mushrooms. Enjoy!

INGREDIENTS

2 portobello mushrooms

2 tablespoons coconut oil, melted

salt (optional)

1 cup basil leaves

1 clove garlic

⅛ cup pine nuts

¼ cup olive oil

black pepper (optional)

salad (your choice of greens)

5 cherry tomatoes, halved

white balsamic vinegar

SUPPLIES

measuring cups and spoon

sharp knife

brush

glass baking dish

food processor

Preheat the oven to 400°F.

Wash the portobello mushrooms to remove excess dirt. Then remove their stems and scoop out their gills.

Use the melted coconut oil to coat the mushrooms and sprinkle lightly with salt if desired.

Place in a glass dish and cook the caps in the oven for about 20 minutes, flipping them halfway through.

While the mushrooms are cooking, place the basil, garlic, and pine nuts in a food processor. Stream in the olive oil. Once smooth, add pepper and salt to taste. This is your pesto sauce!

Place the cooked mushrooms on a plate and drizzle with the pesto sauce.

Add salad greens, cherry tomatoes, and white balsamic vinegar on the side for a nice accompaniment.

Snacks

Blueberry Mango Power Bars

You might have had the chance to try power bars last week if you selected them as part of your Week One snacks. If not, don't worry—these are simple and fast to make. Since this week is all about experimenting, we've provided you with a great variation based on the first power bar recipe.

INGREDIENTS

1¼ cup walnuts

1 cup dried blueberries

½ cup dried mango

½ teaspoon cinnamon powder

⅓ cup egg white protein powder

¼ cup water

SUPPLIES

measuring cups

food processor

large glass dish

Place the walnuts in a food processor and pulse for about 20 seconds, or until granular.

Add the blueberries, mango, cinnamon powder, protein powder, and water, and pulse for about 45 seconds, or until thoroughly combined.

Scoop out the mixture and press into a square or rectangular dish. An 8x8-inch dish makes 10 to 12 half-inch-thick power bars.

Cut the pressed mixture into your desired serving size and place the dish in the refrigerator to set for about an hour.

Serve immediately or keep refrigerated and snack on these bars throughout the week.

Red Pepper Cauliflower Hummus

Yes! Again we're helping you play around with recipes you learned last week. Being able to change up a few core recipes will allow you to experiment with ease and have fun in the process. Red pepper cauliflower hummus happens to be one of our all-time favorite Paleo recipes.

INGREDIENTS

1 red bell pepper, cut in half and seeded

1 head cauliflower, cored and cut into quarter-size florets

2 tablespoons cumin powder

1½ tablespoons coconut oil, melted

4 cloves garlic, halved

½ cup tahini

2 lemons, squeezed

¼ cup water

¼ cup olive oil

5 carrots, for dipping

SUPPLIES

measuring cups and spoons

sharp knife

large mixing bowl

medium oven dish

food processor

Preheat the oven to 450°F.

Place the pepper cut-side down on the oven rack. Roast until skin starts to blister and turn black, about 10 minutes. Remove and let cool.

In a large mixing bowl, mix the cauliflower florets, cumin, coconut oil, and garlic (you may want to use your hands).

Pour the mixture into a baking dish.

Place in the oven to bake for about 30 minutes, or until the cauliflower turns a light golden brown.

Remove from the oven and let cool for about 10 minutes.

Place the cauliflower mixture into a food processor.

Add the red pepper, tahini, lemon juice, and water, and blend until smooth.

Scrape the sides of the processor to ensure the mixture is blended thoroughly.

Stream in the olive oil and pulse for about a minute.

Serve warm or refrigerate and serve chilled within four days.

Use carrots for dipping.

TIP: For a less garlicky version, replace the fresh garlic with garlic powder. This is recommended if you plan to enjoy the hummus over a couple of days.

Teriyaki Jerky

We offered you a traditional version of beef jerky last week, so now it's time to spice it up a little. Have fun with this Paleo-friendly teriyaki jerky!

INGREDIENTS

1 (4- to 5-pound) frozen beef roast

1 (8- to 10-ounce) bottle balsamic vinegar

1 (8 ounce) bottle coconut aminos

1 teaspoon salt

½ cup honey

SUPPLIES

measuring cup

large bowl

aluminum foil

baking sheet

Place the frozen roast out to defrost until the outside rim of the roast is soft but the center is still frozen.

Slice the roast into strips that are about ⅛-inch thick and place the strips in a bowl.

Pour a 50:50 ratio of balsamic vinegar and coconut aminos into the bowl to almost cover the beef strips.

Add the salt and honey, and stir until the marinade coats all of the beef.

Allow the mixture to sit and marinate for at least two hours (overnight in the refrigerator is better if time allows).

Preheat the oven to 190°F.

Place the beef strips onto a foil-lined baking sheet.

Place in the oven to bake and flip about every 30 minutes.

To test if the jerky is done, fold a piece in half and look for white threads. If you see white threads, the jerky is cooked.

Once done, remove the jerky from the oven and allow to cool before serving, or refrigerate and enjoy within 5 days.

TIP: Make sure you cut the jerky thin enough; otherwise, you'll get little, not-so-tasty steaks. Also, having the meat slightly frozen will make it easier to cut. Use a serrated knife and keep hot water running to run your hands under—they will get cold!

Berries or Fruit

Berries or a piece of fruit make a great, quick snack and there are several options to choose from. If you selected this option last week, try experimenting and picking a type of berry or fruit you don't usually consume to gain a variety of nutrients. That said, per last week's comments, stick with berries and fruits that are low on the glycemic index (refer to the *Grocery List*) to make sure you're getting the most out of your Cleanse.

Dried Dates

Dates are always a great option for a Paleo snack; they're also great for kicking a sugar craving. Enjoy up to six dried dates as a morning or afternoon snack.

If you're looking to experiment with dates as a snack, frozen almond butter dates are amazing! Simply cut the date in half, put in about ¼ teaspoon of almond butter, close the date back up, and freeze. Enjoy! One disclaimer though: If you're going with this option, we recommend only having four dates as the almond butter will provide you with an extra boost of energy.

Raw Nuts

Nuts are a fantastic, quick snack, and just like berries or fruit, there are several options to choose from. If you selected this option last week, try experimenting and picking a new type of nut. You can mix it up by choosing almonds, walnuts, cashews, or macadamia nuts that are raw, unsalted, and unsweetened. (Reminder: During the Cleanse we recommend nuts in moderation, at no more than ¼ cup.)

All You Can Eat Vegetable Buffet

Vegetables are wonderful for you. They pack a major nutritional punch, and the best part is that most of them are super lean. If you choose this option as a snack, feel free to indulge and eat as much as you want (as long as you stick to the vegetables on the list!).

Week Two: Let's Experiment

You've decided on your *Meal Plan* and your creative engine is revving. Have fun this week experimenting with new products and recipes. Remember, eating healthy doesn't have to mean eating boring. Truly enjoy Week Two of your journey.

Creativity Rules

There is nothing fun about eating the same thing day in and day out. If you haven't noticed yet, this is not your average cleanse. For one, you actually eat, and second, you get a variety of food. We have crafted all of our recipes, both those in the Cleanse weeks and at the end of the book, to include several variations. This was intentional and essential for a few reasons: First, some of us have food allergies and we simply cannot eat what others can. Second, just because we like something doesn't mean you will, and no one should be restricted to someone else's taste buds. Third, if you master the basic recipe, changing it up when you feel like it won't be an issue.

To further unleash your inner creativity, here are a few things that can easily be switched out to change up a dish:

- seasonings
- vegetables
- fruits
- proteins

Spice Up More Than Your Diet

Another area where some experimentation or change will help increase your Cleanse results is exercise. If you don't exercise regularly, we're not suggesting that you need to start hitting the gym six days a week (though regular exercise is good for you). We are simply saying that incorporating some exercise into your life will help to improve your health, strengthen your bones, and accelerate your Cleanse results. If you are already going to the gym regularly, but typically do the same routine, try introducing another exercise type to activate some muscle groups that you don't normally target.

Switch Up Your Habits

We're changing things up this week, from the foods we eat to the exercise we do. What it really boils down to is changing our habits. Habits are interesting things; most of the time we don't even realize something is a habit. This week is where you really try to start laying down the foundation for some good, healthy habits and start to replace your old, unhealthy ones.

Think about it this way: When you drive to work in the morning, do you usually drive the same way every day? Most likely. What if we told you that there was a better way to go that would cut your commute time by 15 minutes?! You'd be chomping at the bit for us to tell you the new route and yet, despite that enthusiasm, the first week or so might feel strange and uncomfortable. Then suddenly the new route becomes normal and you don't even think about it; you just do it!

That's what you're doing right now. You're adjusting your habits to be healthier and better for you. So keep going with it; pretty soon you won't even think about it, you'll just do it naturally.

Week Two Tips
Always Read the Labels

Experimenting is exciting and fun. However, a very common issue with trying something new is that you might not know everything.

When you go shopping this week, make sure you keep an eye on the food you are purchasing. A closer look at the label will show that many foods hide some not-so-Paleo ingredients. Here are some examples:

Sweet Potato Chips: The store-bought kind is often made with canola oil, which is not Paleo-friendly. Try *Jackson's Honest Chips* for a vegetable oil–free chip alternative.

Almond and/or Coconut Milk: Sometimes refined sugar is added to sweeten these milks. Look closely!

Coconut Yogurt: This usually contains rice starch. Look out!

Gluten-free Anything: Anything gluten-free in the grocery store is commonly made with rice or potato starch. It's a healthier alternative than wheat flour, but it's still not Paleo.

Since most of the foods you will be purchasing will be pure protein and vegetables, you won't need to worry too much about Paleo-unfriendly ingredients. However, for everything else, it's a good idea to keep an eye on the labels. If you do happen to accidentally get something that is not Paleo, don't worry about it; just avoid it the next time you shop.

Relax, It's Not That Scary

We've seen numerous Paleo recipes that take over an hour to make and include ingredients that most people can't even pronounce, let alone know where to purchase. We're here to tell you that Paleo baking and cooking does not need to be overwhelming and it's really not that scary. The recipes in this book have been crafted to be easy and quick to prepare and contain ingredients that can be found at your local grocery or health food store.

Don't Worry about Making a Mistake

Though experimenting is fun and can provide you with fantastic food, there is always the possibility that your food may not turn out quite like you wanted (or intended) it to. Luckily for you, we've provided some great recipes that we have tested countless times to get them just right (and as foolproof as possible). However, if you do decide to go off course—within the realms of the recommended Cleanse foods, of course—and something goes wrong, don't worry about it. There's always tomorrow to try again, and there are also your tried-and-tested Week One recipes for that time or two when things don't go your way. Just have fun and embrace those food disasters as learning experiences. You'll laugh at them in time and they make great stories…we know!

Bye-Bye Cravings

Week Two is when you begin to notice that many of your cravings start to go away. This isn't to say that you'll never have another craving again, but it will start to make saying no to Paleo-unfriendly foods a little bit easier. Enjoy your diminishing cravings; you've earned it through hard work and willpower. If you get a craving this week, don't give in. Pretty soon that craving will be gone for good.

Remember Week One Basics

We gave you a lot of information in Week One and we know that it may have been a lot to remember at once. So, to help refresh your memory and to encourage good habit-building in the early stages of the Cleanse, here's a quick review of the basics necessary for a healthy lifestyle:

- Drink plenty of water.
- Don't keep any temptations around the house, car, office, etc. If you find a candy bar lurking somewhere this week, throw it out immediately.
- Always eat breakfast.
- Expect life to get in the way.
- Eat regularly.
- Chat with your *Accountability Buddy* often.

Biggest Mistake(s)

Of course, when you're doing something like this, you're bound to mess up every now and then. That's quite okay! We had a few instances where we ate something we thought was Paleo and then found out it wasn't. If things like this happen to you, you just need to move forward; don't fret over it. You're changing your lifestyle, and this takes time, mistakes, and learning.

Our biggest mistake came after the Cleanse when we decided to indulge in some Paleo-unfriendly foods. There were a few things we noticed: Eating wheat instantly made each of us feel horrible—gone was the mental clarity and back came the cravings and Camilla's migraines. Wheat was the number-one thing we regretted trying to eat again. Then Melissa gave in to her sugar needs in the form of soda, only the crazy blood sugar spikes and horrendous cravings came right back.

Our biggest mistake boiled down to thinking we could introduce some Paleo-unfriendly foods into our day-to-day diet. This doesn't mean we don't cheat once in a while, but we definitely have to deal with the repercussions of doing so. You're probably going to have to try it yourself to understand, and, if you're anything like us, cheating once will be enough.

Week Two Summary

Fantastic job! You've made it through Week Two of the Paleo Cleanse. You've put in the hard work and it is starting to pay off. As you prepared some new Paleo recipes that were no doubt outside of your comfort zone, you probably realized that Paleo cooking can be delicious without being over-the-top, highly expensive, or time-consuming.

During Week Two you're still adjusting to the Paleo lifestyle. You'll notice that some of your cravings are starting to go away. You may also notice that you might need more food than you originally thought, or maybe you found you don't need as much. Listen to your body—it will always tell you what it needs. As you transition further along with your Ancestral diet, you will become even more in tune with your bodily needs. Make sure to pay attention to them and adjust as you see fit. Our bodies are not all the same—only you can really know what's right for you.

Below is a short summary of what you learned and accomplished this week. Now it's time to get ready for Week Three!

- Eating healthily doesn't have to be plain, redundant, or tasteless. Be creative in the way that you prepare your foods; even a slight change can result in a new discovery.
- Remember to the basics: stay hydrated, eat regularly, and stay in contact with your *Accountability Buddy*.
- Don't limit your creativity to your diet; a change in exercise routine can help you reach new heights in fitness.
- You're starting to switch up your habits, breaking down old ones and making new ones. Pay attention to your body and what it needs.
- Always read your food labels!
- Cooking Paleo meals doesn't have to be scary; it can be easy and enjoyable.
- Don't worry about messing anything up; take everything in stride and remain calm.
- Your cravings are likely starting to disappear, so don't give in now; if you stay strong they'll go away faster!

CHAPTER 14

Paleo Cleanse, Week Three

Welcome to Week Three! You've made it halfway through the Paleo Cleanse and you should be very proud of that fact. This accomplishment should motivate you to keep going. You now only have 16 days left, and it will keep getting easier! The tough part is behind you, and these next two weeks and two days will become more of a routine than a challenge. So keep your commitment to yourself and continue to provide your body with the nourishment it needs to cleanse and revive you.

The next two weeks set the scene for the real changes (and welcome side effects) that the Cleanse delivers. It's worth continuing to experience the difference that Ancestral eating makes in and on your body. Plus, when you get through Week Four, you'll find a tasty, celebratory Paleo dessert recipe waiting for you!

For Week Three, we'll focus on what you might expect your body to go through and introduce new recipes and best practices that apply to this stage in your Cleanse process. Let's get started!

Week Three Meal Plan

Week Three meals build upon the past two weeks but are formulated to maintain a balanced Paleo Diet: Breakfast remains protein-rich and high in fiber; lunch continues to pair refreshing greens with natural fats; dinner still delivers protein, fatty acids, and vegetables; and the snack options remain nutrient-packed for sustenance throughout the day. Of course, the *All You Can Eat Vegetable Buffet* is still available to you as well. Snack on any of those vegetable options whenever you feel the need. Pick and choose what sounds best to you, and as with Week Two, always feel free to include recipes from the previous weeks. Hunger should never be an option, and hydration should remain a top priority.

Week Three Meal Plan Choices

Monday to Sunday Meal Plan Options		
BREAKFAST	Berry Bowl *or* Caprese Baked Egg *or* Breakfast "Sandwich" *or* any Week One or Two Breakfast	**BONUS** All You Can Eat Vegetable Buffet!
SNACK	Date and Orange Bar *or* Sundried Tomato and Basil Hummus *or* Peppered Jerky *or* Stuffed Cold Cuts *or* any Week One or Two Snack	
LUNCH	Chicken Caesar Salad *or* Arugula Berry Salad *or* Deconstructed Tacos *or* any Week One or Two Lunch	
SNACK	Date and Orange Bar *or* Sundried Tomato and Basil Hummus OR Peppered Jerky *or* Stuffed Cold Cuts *or* any Week One or Two Snack	
DINNER	Fajitas *or* Pork Chop and Vegetables *or* Stacked Salmon *or* any Week One or Two Dinner	

Week Three Meal Plan Selection

Fill in your personal *Meal Plan* based on the choices above:

PERSONAL MEAL SELECTION PLAN					
	BREAKFAST	**SNACK**	**LUNCH**	**SNACK**	**DINNER**
MONDAY					
TUESDAY					
WEDNESDAY					
THURSDAY					
FRIDAY					

	BREAKFAST	SNACK	LUNCH	SNACK	DINNER
SATURDAY					
SUNDAY					

Week Three Grocery List

You know the drill—we recommend sticking to organic, grass-fed, free-range, nitrate-free, and GMO-free produce. Happy shopping!

Breakfast

Option 1: Berry Bowl

- berries (blueberries, blackberries, strawberries, and/or raspberries)
- apple
- pear(s)
- coconut milk
- sliced raw almonds

Option 2: Caprese Baked Egg

- coconut oil
- tomato
- dried oregano
- baby spinach leaves
- egg

Option 3: Breakfast "Sandwich"

- coconut oil
- egg
- bacon
- avocado
- black pepper (optional)

Lunch

Option 1: Chicken Caesar Salad

- spinach leaves or spring greens mix
- coconut oil
- chicken breasts
- garlic
- Paleo Caesar Dressing (see page 267)

Option 2: Arugula Berry Salad

- arugula
- strawberries
- sundried tomatoes
- raspberries (fresh or frozen)
- olive oil
- balsamic vinegar
- sliced raw almonds

Option 3: Deconstructed Tacos

- coconut oil
- ground beef
- onion
- sundried tomatoes
- paprika
- shredded lettuce

Dinner

Option 1: Fajitas

- asparagus
- coconut oil
- green bell pepper
- onion
- tahini
- lettuce leaves or coconut wraps
- lemon

Option 2: Pork Chop and Vegetables

- broccoli
- butternut squash
- coconut oil
- pork chop
- paprika

Option 3: Stacked Salmon

- asparagus
- coconut oil
- salmon
- sundried tomatoes
- lemon

Snacks

Option 1: Date and Orange Bars

- walnuts
- dates
- dried apples
- orange

Option 2: Sundried Tomato and Basil Hummus

- cauliflower
- cumin powder

- coconut oil
- garlic (fresh or powdered)
- tahini
- sundried tomatoes
- basil
- lemons
- olive oil
- carrots

Option 3: Peppered Jerky
- frozen beef roast
- balsamic vinegar
- black pepper
- salt

Option 4: Stuffed Cold Cuts
- cold cut meat (roast beef or turkey or ham)
- asparagus or cucumber
- sundried tomatoes
- black pepper

All You Can Eat Vegetable Buffet

- broccoli
- cauliflower
- asparagus
- peppers
- carrots
- cucumber
- eggplant
- celery
- Brussels sprouts

Drink Options

- water
- unsweetened tea
- unsweetened coffee without creamer
- coconut water

As always, if you are unsure of the best place to find any of the above *Grocery List* items, please refer to the *Purchasing Directory* in the back of this book.

Week Three Recipes

Continuing the trend from Weeks One and Two, each of the recipes below makes a single serving, with the exception of the Power Bars, Hummus, and Jerky, which will provide you with four to five servings. If you have found that preparing your weekly meals is best done in advance, simply multiply the quantity in the recipes below by the number of times you plan to enjoy each meal this week.

Breakfast

Berry Bowl

A fiber-rich, nutrient-filled burst of morning flavor, this breakfast bowl is so tasty you won't believe it's so good for you.

INGREDIENTS

¼ cup berries

1 apple, cored and chopped

1 pear, cored and chopped (if out of season, use 2 apples)

¼ cup coconut milk

1 tablespoon sliced almonds

measuring cups

sharp knife

food processor

Place the berries, apple, and pear in a food processor and pulse until chopped.

Add the coconut milk and continue to pulse for another 1 to 2 minutes, until the mixture is smooth.

Pour into a breakfast bowl and sprinkle with almonds.

Serve chilled.

Caprese Baked Egg

The yolk in this gourmet baked egg dish provides you with a boost of protein, iron, vitamin A, and vitamin C to start your day right.

INGREDIENTS

¼ teaspoon coconut oil

1 thick slice fresh tomato

¼ teaspoon dried oregano

3 to 4 fresh baby spinach leaves

1 egg

SUPPLIES

measuring cups

sharp knife

small ramekin

Preheat the oven to 450°F.

Grease a small ramekin with coconut oil.

Place the slice of tomato at the bottom of the ramekin and sprinkle with oregano.

Top the tomato with spinach.

Crack the egg on top of the spinach.

Place in the oven for 11 to 13 minutes for a soft yolk, or 13 to 15 minutes for a hard yolk.

Remove from the oven and serve hot.

Breakfast "Sandwich"

This morning delight gives a Paleo twist to the popular breakfast sandwich. It is flavorful and full of healthy fats and proteins to power your morning.

INGREDIENTS

¼ teaspoon coconut oil

1 egg

1 strip bacon

½ avocado, sliced in half

black pepper (optional)

SUPPLIES

measuring spoon

sharp knife

aluminum foil

baking tray

small ramekin

Preheat the oven to 425°F.

Line a baking tray with foil.

Grease a small ramekin with coconut oil.

Crack the egg into the ramekin.

Slice the bacon strip in half and place on the foil-lined baking sheet.

Place the baking sheet and the ramekin in the oven for about 10 minutes for a soft yolk and soft bacon, or about 12 minutes for a hard yolk and crispy bacon.

Remove from the oven and allow to cool for about 2 minutes.

On a plate, place one half of the strip of the bacon and top with one slice of avocado.

Remove the egg from the baking dish and place on top of the avocado.

Sprinkle with black pepper if desired.

Complete the sandwich by placing the second piece of avocado on top of the egg, followed by the second piece of bacon.

Enjoy while warm.

Lunch

Chicken Caesar Salad

Delicately balancing fresh greens and grilled chicken, this lunch option is light yet satisfying and offers a variety of nutrients, including omega-3 fatty acids, selenium, and vitamin C.

INGREDIENTS

2 cups spinach or spring greens mix

1 tablespoon coconut oil

¼ pound chicken breasts, sliced thinly

1 tablespoon garlic, crushed

Paleo Caesar Dressing (see page 267)

SUPPLIES

measuring cups and spoons

sharp knife

medium bowl

medium sauté pan

Place the greens in a medium bowl.

In a medium sauté pan, melt the coconut oil over medium heat.

Add the chicken breast strips and the garlic and cook over medium heat until the chicken is well-done.

Once cooked, place the chicken strips on the bed of greens.

Pour Paleo Caesar dressing over the chicken.

Arugula Berry Salad

Fresh, sweet, and antioxidant-rich, this berry salad delivers vitamins, minerals, and fructose to give you energy for the afternoon.

INGREDIENTS

2 cups arugula

½ cup strawberries, sliced

¼ cup sundried tomatoes, sliced thinly

¼ cup raspberries (fresh or frozen)

2 tablespoons olive oil

2 tablespoons balsamic vinegar

2 tablespoons raw almonds, sliced

SUPPLIES

measuring cups and spoons

sharp knife

medium mixing bowl

food processor

shaker

In a mixing bowl, toss the arugula, strawberries, and sundried tomatoes.

In a food processor, puree the raspberries until they are liquid.

Pour the raspberry puree into a small bowl or shaker and add the olive oil and balsamic vinegar. Mix or shake until well combined.

Pour the dressing mixture over the salad, top with almonds, and serve chilled or at room temperature.

Deconstructed Tacos

A balance of hot and refreshing, this grain-free take on the traditional taco makes for a delicious lunch high in protein, natural fats, fiber, and antioxidants.

INGREDIENTS

1 teaspoon coconut oil

¼ pound ground beef

¼ cup chopped onion

¼ cup sundried tomatoes

1 teaspoon paprika

1½ cups shredded lettuce

SUPPLIES

measuring cups and spoon

sharp knife

medium sauté pan

In a medium sauté pan, melt the coconut oil over medium heat and then add the beef.

Stirring often, let brown for about 4 minutes before adding the onion, tomatoes, and paprika.

Once the meat has browned (typically after about 10 minutes), remove from the heat.

On a dinner plate, spread the lettuce and top with the beef taco mixture.

Enjoy while the meat is hot.

Dinner

Fajitas

A light and tasty snack, this Mexican-inspired dish takes
a Paleo turn, combining natural fibers, oils, and minerals
to provide you with a well-balanced dinner.

INGREDIENTS

¼ pound asparagus, ends cut off

1 teaspoon coconut oil

½ green bell pepper, sliced into strips

½ onion, sliced into strips

1 teaspoon tahini

2 lettuce leaves or 1 coconut wrap

½ lemon

measuring cups

sharp knife

large pot

medium sauté pan

Bring water to a boil in a pot and add the asparagus.

In a medium sauté pan, melt the coconut oil over medium heat and then add the green pepper and onion, browning slightly.

Remove the asparagus from the pot when tender and add to the green pepper and onion mix.

Add the tahini to the mixture, stir briefly and allow to sit for another minute or two.

On a dinner plate, place your choice of wrap and fill with the fajita mixture.

Top with freshly squeezed lemon juice and serve while warm.

Pork Chop and Vegetables

This hearty meal disguises zinc, potassium, and plenty of vitamins in a comforting, protein-rich dish.

INGREDIENTS

¼ pound broccoli, chopped

¼ pound butternut squash, chopped

1 teaspoon coconut oil

¼ pound pork chop

½ teaspoon paprika

SUPPLIES

measuring cups

sharp knife

medium pot

medium sauté pan

strainer

Bring water to a boil in a pot and add the broccoli and butternut squash.

In a medium sauté pan, melt the coconut oil over medium heat and then add the pork chop.

Cook both the pork and the vegetables, each for 12 to 15 minutes, turning the pork every few minutes.

Once the vegetables are tender, strain them and arrange on a dinner plate.

Once the pork is well-done, place it alongside the vegetables.

Sprinkle paprika over the vegetables and enjoy while hot.

Stacked Salmon

Not only does salmon provide essential fatty acids, it's abundant in vitamins B and D, making this decadent dish a joy for you and your body.

INGREDIENTS

¼ pound asparagus, ends cut off

1 tablespoon coconut oil

¼ pound salmon fillet

¼ cup sundried tomatoes, sliced into strips

1 lemon

SUPPLIES

measuring cups

sharp knife

large pot

medium sauté pan

Bring water to a boil in a large pot and add the asparagus. Cook until tender, then strain and set aside.

In a medium sauté pan, melt the coconut oil over medium heat and then add the salmon.

Cook for about 5 minutes, flip the fillet, and continue to cook for another 5 to 10 minutes.

Once fully cooked, plate the salmon and top with sundried tomatoes.

Place the asparagus on top of the sundried tomatoes.

Squeeze lemon juice over the salmon stack and serve hot.

Snacks

Date and Orange Bars

A great snack to carry with you on the go, these bars are
fiber-rich, high in omega-3 fatty acids, and flavored with
natural citrus for that extra boost of vitamin C.

INGREDIENTS

1¼ cup walnuts

1 cup dates, chopped

½ cup dried apples

grated zest of 1 orange

1 tablespoon water

2 tablespoons freshly squeezed orange juice

SUPPLIES

measuring cups and spoon

food processor

large glass dish

Place the walnuts in a food processor and pulse for about 20 seconds, or
until granular.

Add the dates and pulse for another minute before adding the apples,
orange zest, water, and orange juice. Pulse for about 45 seconds, or until
thoroughly combined.

Scoop out the mixture and press into a square or rectangular dish. An
8x8-inch dish makes 10 to 12 half-inch-thick power bars.

Cut the pressed mixture into your desired serving size and place the dish
in the refrigerator to set for about an hour.

Serve immediately or keep refrigerated and snack on these bars
throughout the week.

Sundried Tomato and Basil Hummus

As we continue to get creative and build upon the basics, this variation of the original Cauliflower Hummus recipe makes for a gourmet treat.

INGREDIENTS

1 head cauliflower, cored and cut into quarter-size florets

2 tablespoons cumin powder

1½ tablespoons coconut oil, melted

4 cloves garlic, halved

½ cup tahini

5 sundried tomatoes, sliced

4 fresh basil leaves

2 lemons, squeezed

¼ cup water

¼ cup olive oil

5 carrots, for dipping

SUPPLIES

measuring cups

sharp knife

large mixing bowl

oven-safe dish

food processor

Preheat the oven to 450°F.

In a large mixing bowl, mix the cauliflower florets, cumin, coconut oil, and garlic (you may want to use your hands).

Pour the mixture into a baking dish.

Place in the oven to bake for 30 minutes, or until the cauliflower turns light golden brown.

Remove from the oven and let cool for about 10 minutes.

Place the cauliflower mixture into a food processor.

Add the tahini, sundried tomatoes, basil, lemon juice, and water, and blend until smooth.

Scrape the sides of the processor to ensure the mixture is blended thoroughly.

Stream in the olive oil and pulse for about a minute.

Serve warm or refrigerate and serve chilled within four days.

Use carrots for dipping.

TIP: For a less garlicky version, replace the fresh garlic with garlic powder. This is recommended if you plan to enjoy the hummus over several days.

Peppered Jerky

Another variation of the Week One classic, this snack rivals store-bought jerky and remains soy- and wheat-free.

INGREDIENTS

1 (4- to 5-pound) frozen beef roast

1 (8- to 10-ounce) bottle balsamic vinegar

2 tablespoons black pepper, divided

1 teaspoon salt

SUPPLIES

measuring cups

sharp knife

deep bowl

aluminum foil

baking sheet

Place the frozen roast out to defrost until the outside rim of the roast is soft but the center is still frozen.

Slice the roast into ⅛-inch-thick strips and place the strips in a bowl.

Pour enough balsamic vinegar into the bowl to almost cover the beef strips.

Sprinkle with 1 tablespoon black pepper and salt and stir until the marinade coats all the beef.

Allow the mixture to sit and marinate for at least two hours (overnight in the refrigerator is best, if time allows).

Preheat the oven to 190°F.

Place the beef strips onto a foil-lined baking sheet.

Sprinkle with the other tablespoon of black pepper.

Place in the oven to bake and flip about every 30 minutes.

To test if the jerky is done, fold a piece in half and look for white threads. If you see the white threads the jerky is cooked.

Once you've confirmed it's done, remove the jerky from the oven and allow to cool before serving, or refrigerate and enjoy within five days.

TIP: Make sure you cut the jerky thin enough; otherwise you'll get little, not-so-tasty steaks. Also, having the meat slightly frozen will make it easier to cut. Use a serrated knife and keep hot water running to run your hands under—they will get cold!

Stuffed Cold Cuts

This quick and easy snack is high in protein and dietary fiber. Plus, asparagus is composed of over 90 percent water and helps to equalize the natural sodium found in meat.

INGREDIENTS

1 slice cold cut meat

1 cooked asparagus spear or slice of cucumber

1 thin strip sundried tomato

black pepper

SUPPLIES

sharp knife

toothpicks (optional)

Fold open the slice of cold cut meat and place the asparagus or cucumber in the center.

Top with the sundried tomato and sprinkle with black pepper.

Roll the cold cut meat into a wrap and leave as is or pierce in place with a toothpick.

Serve chilled.

Berries or Fruit, Dried Dates, Raw Nuts and All You Can Eat Vegetable Buffet

These snack staples remain consistent from the previous weeks. Please visit Chapters 12 and 13 to review information about these great snack choices.

Week Three: Routine Kicks In

The end of Week Two and the close of the halfway mark on the Cleanse is the turning point for both your body and your mind. Week Three is where routines kicks in and the benefits of the Cleanse begin to unfold.

Week Three is all about getting comfortable, settling in to your new dietary lifestyle and enjoying the newfound benefits it has on your body. This is when the switch happens, from longing for carbohydrates and refined sugar products to realizing how much better it feels to eat well. This is also when your cravings should diminish almost entirely and the true benefits of the Cleanse begin to show. Don't think about it too much or let your mind interfere with your newfound method.

Continue exactly as you have been and allow your transformation to happen without concerning yourself with it. Focus only on the routine of grocery shopping days, meal preparation, regular snacking, and healthy hydration. Stick with this method that got you through the first two weeks, and you'll finish three-quarters of your Paleo Cleanse before you know it.

Week Three Tips

This third week takes you to Day 21—the date that signifies the potential for a changed habit. After 21 consecutive days of sticking to something new, the likelihood of continuing past that date becomes great. Considering that, this week is very important. You have two weeks of Paleo Cleanse experience, so be disciplined with yourself this week and use the following tips to help solidify the habit of healthy eating.

Mix Up Your Snacks

As you refill your snack stash, you may want to consider mixing it up a little: If you have been eating almonds, try a mix of almonds and walnuts; if you have been eating Granny Smith apples, try Fuji or Red Delicious. The different food varieties and colors have different nutrients to offer, and at this point in the Cleanse, you are beyond any serious cravings, so switching up food choices should be easier than ever.

Getting Comfortable Doesn't Mean Getting Lazy

You've done the drill for two weeks now, so at this point the little things have become second nature. Replenishing your snack bag for on-the-go nibbling and refilling your water bottle were once something you had to think about to remember, but now they just come naturally. If you think it's suddenly okay to skip a cooking day or not bring a Power Bar to work, don't do it! While your body is still adjusting to its new diet and is much healthier and happier than before, the proper nourishment and continued dedication is still necessary to completing your Paleo Cleanse successfully.

As you work your way through Week Three, remember that it never pays to cut corners. It's very typical in life to start cutting corners, lose momentum, and leave things unpolished or undone as soon as you begin to feel comfortable with what you are doing. This is a recipe for failure and a trait of the unsuccessful. It's like the story of Apple when they decided to do away with Steve Jobs; if you stop concerning yourself with doing the very best, you stop being the very best. This Cleanse is only 30 days of your life—give it all you've got and keep on going!

Avoid Complication

If you're feeling good about your progress and you're comfortable with the Cleanse *Meal Plans*, it might be tempting to get overly complicated. It would be great to have peppered jerky to snack on for Monday and teriyaki for Tuesday, etc., but be realistic with your time and ability to keep on track if you choose to go to this extent.

Even once we had reached Week Three in our Cleanse journey, we didn't have the time to cook a unique recipe each day. We still picked a few of our favorites out of the recipe options, prepared them on our designated cooking day(s), and then enjoyed them the remainder of the week. This particularly applies to the snack options.

Making two snack options, like we did, is perfectly good enough; if you can do even more than that, do it! We invite you to get comfortable in your creativity and make the Cleanse truly personalized to you. But in doing so, just be careful that you don't end up biting off more than you can chew. Whatever you choose to make and however you design your Week Three *Meal Plan*, make sure it's manageable for you. Ease and convenience are the keys to continued success at this stage in the Cleanse. Always have enough of the basics on hand to get you through the week, and then have fun experimenting.

Stick to Your Grocery Day(s)

Sometimes when routine kicks in it's easy to slack off. You think you have it down pat and you'll just do it tomorrow. Don't! Pushing anything off to tomorrow is not a good idea (we know!). If your designated grocery day worked for you in Weeks One and Two, stick to shopping on that same day this week, too. Keep everything as consistent as possible and your third week will go by as smoothly as can be.

Eating Out Still Isn't a Good Option

As the *Meal Plans* get more interesting week after week, you may start to wonder whether eating out is a viable option. We know how tempting it is after two straight weeks of preparing three meals a day, plus snacks, at home. You probably feel like you deserve a break, and truthfully, you do. Unfortunately, eating out is still not a great solution, and you should continue to restrict doing so as much as possible. If you're going to eat out—try to keep it Paleo.

Results Don't Mean All Is Said and Done

By now, there is a good chance you are enjoying some welcome side effects of Paleo eating. Maybe you've noticed a decline in recurring headaches, an improvement in your mood, and a sounder night's sleep. You should also be friendly and accepting of your bathroom scale and may well like what it's showing you. With weight loss being a definite reality at this stage of the Paleo Cleanse, you could have dropped a couple of pounds, with your body fat percentage a few points lower. You feel healthier, lighter, and happier. It's almost worth celebrating with a cupcake, right? Wrong!

We know the saying goes that it's best to give up when you're ahead, but this is not one of those cases. The truth is, you're not yet ahead—you're about to reach the peak and fly. It takes time to allow your body to truly cleanse from the inside out. Think of this stage in the Cleanse as the harvest season. Continue to sow and sow and sow! By committing to a high-quality diet, you've already taken half the action. If you give up now, you'll only get half the results. Just hold on and keep at it, and you will soon reap the whole reward.

Despondency Isn't Your Friend

If you happen to be on the other end of the spectrum and have yet to feel anything significantly different despite your dedication to the Cleanse—don't get down about it. You're not doing anything wrong and your efforts are not futile; it just means that your body adjusts at a different speed.

It is no doubt frustrating to try so hard and not feel any change, but know this: When you change anything you do, you change the outcome you create. It may take time (and Week Three might just be your week), but it will happen. Stay committed, keep motivated, and press on.

As always, we're here to help, and so is the rest of the wonderful Paleo community. Join us at ThePaleoPact.com whenever you feel the need for some Paleo Cleanse motivation.

Consider It an Investment

As your grocery expense has climbed and your time in the kitchen has quadrupled, you may start to question if this is all worth it. Yes, it is! We know that it's hard to justify at first and, trust us, we've had our moments of receipt-inflicted horror. But what it comes down to is this: Your health is all you've got.

Without your health, you have literally nothing. Your health is the single most valuable thing you possess, and it's worth the time to maintain it. Choose to have the mentality that your health is your greatest investment, because it truly is.

See the Glass as Half Full

From Day 1 we emphasized the importance of attitude, and as you proceed through your final two weeks this is more important than ever. We've covered a lot in this chapter about some common causes of failure: getting lazy and feeling despondent over lack of early results. We know that you're not going to fall for either of those two obstacles and that you will hurdle along through the next two weeks of your Cleanse journey.

Rather than viewing your current stage in the process as merely halfway through, let your mid-month milestone ignite even more passion toward your commitment—you're halfway done! You have already proven that you have the willpower it takes to succeed, and now there is a light at the end of the tunnel, so keep moving forward.

You're Important, Not Selfish

It may sound selfish, but really, taking care of You is the most important thing you can do. Without a state of health, you can't properly take care of anyone else. Plus, the example you are setting for your family, your friends, and even your coworkers is not only admirable, it's inspiring. The actions you have taken to get where you are now speaks volumes about your personal commitment to health and illustrates your ability to demonstrate willpower and productive discipline. We're proud of you and we hope you are very proud of yourself, too.

Motivate Yourself with a Finish Line Reward

We are huge fans of *Self-Created Challenges* and *Reward Programs*. We are firm believers in the power of earned celebration. We encourage you to implement this in your life and, if you haven't done so already, plan a reward for when you complete Week Four of the Paleo Cleanse.

What is a *Self-Created Challenge?* It is a goal you set for yourself that is well-defined, well-planned, and has a clear end, such as running a 5km race in under 30 minutes within two months. In essence, the Paleo Cleanse is a challenge with an objective of good health. It has a clear timeline, a clear plan of action, and a clear objective.

What is a *Reward Program?* A reward program is the way to make a challenge interesting. It adds an incentive to look forward to once you complete the goal. Perhaps you told yourself you could have a new pair of running shoes if you complete the run in under 30 minutes, as an example. In relation to the Cleanse, rather than merely checking off the last day on your *Cleanse Calendar*, a scheduled reward offers a celebration to look forward to.

The concept of celebrating your achievements is an ancient one, but something that is underappreciated and underpracticed in our modern times. We remember to celebrate birthdays (usually!) and major life events such as weddings and graduations, but we so often forget to celebrate the little things. The Cleanse may be considered a small accomplishment in comparison, but really it's a life-changing event—it's improving your health. By celebrating, you reward yourself for completing your goals and you grant yourself well-deserved enjoyment, which promotes productivity and happiness, and also encourages you to continue your personal progress by creating a new challenge. Maybe the motivation from completing your Paleo Cleanse will encourage you to continue your Paleo journey. (We'll address this further in Chapter 17.)

Just choose your reward wisely. To provide the motivation it should, the reward must be something that you really enjoy or want. If you love getting massages, schedule one for the day you will be finished with the Cleanse. If there is a pair of shoes you've been wanting, promise yourself that you will buy them after Day 30. If it's a weekend getaway you desire, book it now. Whatever it is (and it doesn't need to be expensive), it should be meaningful to you; pick something that will either provide you with wonderful memories or that will serve as a constant reminder of what you accomplished.

Week Three Summary

Three weeks down! You're a whole lot further down your personal path toward perfect health. Give yourself a huge pat on the back. Whether you feel it yet or not, your body and every cell within is thanking you. Keep up with the following Week Three Tips:

- Stay focused and apply the best practices you learned during Weeks One and Two.
- For continued results, keep it simple and stick to your previous grocery shopping and designated cooking days.

(Remember to take the *Grocery List* with you to the store for added convenience.)

- Keep doing what works, crystallize your actions into habits, avoid complication, and prevent yourself from becoming lazy.
- Check your snack stash and refill it as necessary; continue to refrain from eating out.
- If you're already seeing great results, hold on longer—you're about to enjoy more; if you have yet to experience results, don't get despondent—your time lies ahead.
- Keep your attitude in check, let positivity reign, and choose to view the monetary spending and time commitment as an investment in your health and your future.
- Motivate yourself with a reward to look forward to once you complete the full 30 days.

CHAPTER 15

Paleo Cleanse, Week Four

Welcome to Week Four of the Paleo Cleanse! You're in the home stretch and only a week away from completing your Paleo Cleanse. At this point you've learned a lot about the Paleo lifestyle and are probably hitting your stride and getting the hang of Paleo cooking. Most likely, you have also begun to notice the difference it makes in your life. The great news is that it keeps getting easier and better, so let's dive straight into Week Four.

Stay Prepared to Finish Strong

By now you're accustomed to cooking days and know which Paleo snacks require little to no preparation. Make sure to have plenty of these on hand and stick with your cooking days. You're so close to being finished; stay prepared and you'll stay strong!

Listen to Your Body and Prepare for Post-Cleanse Living

Everyone's body is completely different, which also means that we each have a unique set of needs. The best person to determine what your body needs is you, so this week, focus on what your body is telling you. Monitor yourself and ask questions like: Do I feel like I'm getting enough food? Do I feel energized? Do I really need caffeine? Do I feel rested enough? Depending on your answers, you may need to adjust your food portions and the types of food you're consuming (within the realm of the Cleanse, of course), so that you have the appropriate diet to fuel your lifestyle.

You should also use this week to determine what types of Paleo foods you really like, which ones provide you with a lot of energy, and which ones you wouldn't miss. While you complete this week, spend time truly observing these preferences and take mental notes (or better yet, jot down your findings in a journal). Once you have completed your Cleanse and begin transitioning into a post-Cleanse lifestyle of your choice, you will be able to incorporate this book's weekly and bonus recipes (Chapter 23) into your everyday diet.

Prepare for Your Celebration

You've put a lot of time into this Cleanse and you deserve to treat yourself. You picked your reward last week, and now it's time to ensure you are prepared for the special something you chose. Remember, this can be as simple or as grand as you want. You could even celebrate in the literal sense by throwing a Paleo Cleanse party and sharing some of the great foods you've learned to master over the past few weeks! You can find Paleo-friendly party recipes at ThePaleoPact.com.

Get excited by looking ahead, but also hone in and focus on Week Four of your journey. Stay committed during your last full week and really have fun with it.

Week Four Meal Plan

The options this week are delicious and easy to prepare to make sure that you have no excuses for not finishing your Cleanse. As always you can also use recipes from the previous weeks, so your options are now quite varied. Remember, though, to purchase your groceries and prepare your chosen meals in advance whenever possible. While you may be getting comfortable with Paleo cooking and feel your options are endless, preparing your meals early will give you one less excuse to cheat and will help to alleviate stress.

Week Four Meal Plan Choices

Monday to Sunday Meal Plan Options		
BREAKFAST	Pear and Pork Sausage *or* Green Smoothie *or* Huevos Rancheros *or* any Week One, Two, or Three Breakfast	**BONUS** All You Can Eat Vegetable Buffet!
SNACK	Cranberry Zest Power Bar *or* Jalapeño Cauliflower Hummus *or* Spicy Jerky *or* any Week One, Two, or Three Snack	
LUNCH	Beet Arugula Salad *or* Nicoise Salad *or* Chicken Burger and Cauliflower Mash *or* any Week One, Two, or Three Lunch	
SNACK	Cranberry Zest Power Bar *or* Jalapeño Cauliflower Hummus *or* Spicy Jerky *or* any Week One, Two, or Three Snack	
DINNER	Stuffed Chicken Breast *or* Steak and Vegetables *or* Truffle Cauliflower Risotto *or* any Week One, Two, or Three Dinner	

Week Four Meal Plan Selection

Fill in your personal *Meal Plan* based on the choices above:

PERSONAL MEAL PLAN SELECTION

	BREAKFAST	SNACK	LUNCH	SNACK	DINNER
MONDAY					
TUESDAY					
WEDNESDAY					
THURSDAY					
FRIDAY					

	BREAKFAST	SNACK	LUNCH	SNACK	DINNER
SATURDAY					
SUNDAY					

Week Four Grocery List

As always, we recommend sticking to organic, grass-fed, free-range, nitrate-free, and GMO-free produce.

Breakfast

Option 1: Pear and Pork Sausage

- pork sausage
- pear
- honey

Option 2: Green Smoothie

- banana
- orange
- spinach
- honey
- almond milk
- egg white protein powder (optional)
- ice

Option 3: Huevos Rancheros

- coconut oil
- yellow onion
- tomatoes
- green chilies
- chili powder
- cumin powder
- salt
- black pepper
- eggs

Lunch

Option 1: Beet Arugula Salad

- beets
- walnuts
- orange
- olive oil
- balsamic vinegar
- honey
- salt
- arugula

Option 2: Nicoise Salad

- romaine lettuce
- tomatoes
- tuna
- hardboiled eggs
- olives
- Paleo Caesar Dressing (see page 267)

Option 3: Chicken Burger with Cauliflower Mash

- cauliflower
- coconut oil

- cumin powder
- almond milk
- ground chicken
- salt
- black pepper
- red onion
- cilantro

Dinner

Option 1: Stuffed Chicken Breast
- spinach
- coconut oil
- bacon
- chicken breast
- salt
- black pepper

Option 2: Steak and Veggies
- vegetables (your choice from the *All You Can Eat Vegetable Buffet*)
- coconut oil
- steak
- spices (your choice of salt, pepper, dried oregano, or any other spice you enjoy)

Option 3: Truffle Cauliflower Risotto
- vegetables (your choice from the *All You Can Eat Vegetable Buffet*)
- cauliflower
- mushrooms
- salt
- black pepper
- avocado
- coconut milk
- garlic

Snacks

Option 1: Cranberry Zest Power Bars

- walnuts
- dried cranberries
- oranges
- egg white protein powder (optional)

Option 2: Jalapeño Cauliflower Hummus

- jalapeño
- cauliflower
- cumin powder
- coconut oil
- garlic (fresh or powdered)
- tahini
- lemons
- olive oil
- carrots

Option 3: Spicy Jerky

- frozen beef roast
- balsamic vinegar
- coconut aminos
- jalapeño
- red pepper flakes
- salt
- honey

All You Can Eat Vegetable Buffet

- broccoli
- cauliflower
- asparagus
- peppers

- carrots
- cucumber
- eggplant
- celery
- Brussels sprouts

Drink Options

- water
- unsweetened tea
- unsweetened coffee without creamer
- coconut water

If you are not sure of the best place to find any of the above items, refer to the *Purchasing Directory* in the back of this book.

Week Four Recipes

Each of the recipes below makes a single serving, with the exception of the Power Bars, Hummus and Jerky, which will provide you with four to five servings. If you are preparing your Week Four meals in advance, simply multiply the quantity in the below recipes by the number of times you plan to enjoy each recipe during the week.

Breakfast

Pear and Pork Sausage

Breakfast sausage is a staple and will keep you powered throughout your morning. Try switching out the pear with apple if you want to experiment a little.

INGREDIENTS

1 large pork sausage

¼ pear

1 teaspoon honey

measuring spoon

sharp knife

aluminum foil

baking sheet

Preheat the oven to 450°F.

Slice the pork sausage in half the long way, being careful to keep it attached on one end.

Slice the pear into thin strips and place the slices on top of the pork sausage.

Drizzle with honey.

Close the sausage halves to form a sandwich and place on a foil-lined baking sheet.

Place in the oven and cook for 10 to 15 minutes, or until well-done.

Green Smoothie

Don't let the green color of this smoothie freak you out—it tastes delicious! This smoothie is packed with natural nutrients to help sustain your energy level throughout the day. It's also incredibly easy to make.

1 banana

1 orange, squeezed

1 cup spinach leaves

2 tablespoons honey

⅓ cup almond milk

⅓ cup egg white protein powder (optional)

5 ice cubes

SUPPLIES

measuring cups

sharp knife

blender

to-go cup

Place the banana, orange juice, spinach, honey, almond milk, protein powder, and ice in a blender.

Blend until smooth.

Pour into your to-go container and you're ready to walk out the door!

Huevos Rancheros

Huevos Rancheros is a delicious and fun breakfast option that we've varied slightly to make Paleo-friendly. This dish is a great way to spice up your morning. It's also a great way to trick your loved ones into eating healthily with you!

INGREDIENTS

2 tablespoons coconut oil, divided

½ yellow onion, diced

2 large tomatoes, diced

½ cup diced green chilies

2 tablespoons chili powder

1 tablespoon cumin powder

½ teaspoon salt

½ teaspoon black pepper

2 eggs

SUPPLIES

measuring cup and spoons

sharp knife

2 medium sauté pans

Melt 1 tablespoon of coconut oil in a sauté pan over medium heat.

Add the diced onion, tomatoes, chilies, chili powder, cumin, salt, and pepper to the pan, and heat until the onions and tomatoes are cooked thoroughly and are soft.

In another sauté pan, melt the other tablespoon of coconut oil over medium-high heat.

Crack the eggs and place them in the second frying pan to cook. Cook the eggs however you'd like; traditionally, they are done over-easy.

Place the eggs on a plate and cover with the onion, tomato, and chili mixture.

Enjoy while hot.

Lunch

Beet Arugula Salad

Beets are fantastic vegetables packed full of nutrients. In this recipe we'll show you how to make a flavorful, healthy salad that is sure to make your taste buds and cells happy!

INGREDIENTS

3 beets, peeled and cubed

¼ cup walnuts

1 orange, squeezed

2 tablespoons olive oil

2 tablespoons balsamic vinegar

1 tablespoon honey

½ teaspoon salt

arugula

SUPPLIES

measuring cup and spoons

sharp knife

peeler

medium pot

small sauté pan

small mixing bowl

whisk

Pour water into a medium pot and bring to a boil.

Add the beets cubes to the boiling water. Boil for about 20 minutes, or until you can poke a skewer through them.

In a sauté pan over medium heat, toast the walnuts until you can smell the nut aroma in the air. (You don't want to burn them, so keep an eye on them and toss them regularly.)

In a mixing bowl, add the orange juice, olive oil, balsamic vinegar, honey, and salt. Whisk until well combined. This is your homemade dressing!

Arrange the arugula on a plate and top with the beets and walnuts before drizzling with the dressing.

Nicoise Salad

This salad is the perfect Paleo-approved antipasti. On the Cleanse we list it as a lunch option; post-Cleanse you might enjoy serving it as a delicious dinner appetizer. This is also a salad that you can adjust to fit your taste buds, so feel free to experiment with different ingredients (within the Cleanse list, of course).

INGREDIENTS
romaine lettuce

1 cup cherry tomatoes, halved

1 can tuna

2 hardboiled eggs, quartered

½ cup olives

Paleo Caesar Dressing (see page 267)

SUPPLIES
measuring cups

sharp knife

On a plate, arrange the bed of lettuce.

In sections on top of the lettuce, place the tomatoes, tuna, eggs, and olives.

Lightly drizzle with Paleo Caesar dressing.

It's that easy. Enjoy!

Chicken Burger with Cauliflower Mash

This meal is delicious, well-rounded, and filling; it's also super-lean, which is sure to help you with your Cleanse goals this final week.

INGREDIENTS

½ head cauliflower

1 tablespoon coconut oil, melted

2 tablespoons cumin powder, divided

¼ cup almond milk

½ pound ground chicken

1 teaspoon salt

1 teaspoon black pepper

¼ red onion, diced

¼ cup cilantro, chopped

SUPPLIES

measuring cups and spoons

sharp knife

medium mixing bowl

medium baking dish

food processor

grill

Preheat the oven to 450°F.

Core the cauliflower and cut into ¼-inch florets.

In a mixing bowl, gently mix the cauliflower with the coconut oil and 1 tablespoon of cumin powder.

Place the cauliflower mix in a baking dish and place in the oven for 20 to 30 minutes, or until you can poke a skewer through the cauliflower.

Add the cauliflower mixture to a food processor, along with the almond milk, and blend until smooth.

Preheat the grill to medium-high heat.

In a mixing bowl, combine the chicken, salt, pepper, other tablespoon of cumin powder, diced red onion, and chopped cilantro. Form into patties.

Grill the patties for about 10 minutes, or until fully cooked.

Plate alongside the cauliflower mash and enjoy while warm.

Dinner

Stuffed Chicken Breast

A light but incredibly filling dinner that is sure to make everyone happy; what can we say—it has bacon! This can be served standalone or with your choice of vegetables from the *All You Can Eat Vegetable Buffet.*

INGREDIENTS
1 cup of raw spinach

1 tablespoon coconut oil

4 slices cooked bacon

2 chicken breasts

salt

black pepper

SUPPLIES
measuring cups

sharp knife

2 medium sauté pans

medium glass baking dish

Preheat the oven to 375°F.

Place the spinach and coconut oil in a sauté pan and cook over medium heat until the spinach has wilted.

Place the bacon in a sauté pan and cook over medium-high heat until desired finish, then remove from the heat and drain the fat.

Chop the bacon strips into small pieces and mix with the spinach.

Slice into the side of the chicken breast, making small pockets. Fill these pockets with the bacon and spinach mixture, then sprinkle with salt and pepper.

Place the stuffed chicken breast into a glass baking dish and place it in the oven.

Cook until well-done, about 45 minutes.

Remove from the oven and serve hot.

Steak and Veggies

This is your dish, made your way. Feel free to choose any grass-fed steak cut and Paleo-friendly vegetables (from the *All You Can Eat Vegetable Buffet*). If you're not feeling like having steak you can also substitute the protein with fish or chicken.

INGREDIENTS

vegetables (your choice from the *All You Can Eat Vegetable Buffet*)

1 tablespoon coconut oil

½ pound steak cut of your choice

spices (your choice of salt, pepper, dried oregano, or any other spice you enjoy)

SUPPLIES

measuring spoon

sharp knife

Aluminum foil

grill or medium pot and medium sauté pan

This is your show, but we recommend grilling because it provides great taste and it's super easy. The vegetables can also be grilled. You can wrap them in foil with a little coconut oil and simply set them alongside your steak.

If you choose to cook on the stove-top, bring your vegetables to a boil in a medium pot and cook your steak over medium heat in a tablespoon of melted coconut oil.

Spice as you desire and enjoy as you prefer.

Truffle Cauliflower Risotto

Risotto is a common favorite; unfortunately it's not exactly Paleo-friendly. That's why we've come up with a great substitute that will let you indulge without any of the guilt. When you're done with the Cleanse you can consider adding a little grass-fed cheese to enhance the flavor of the dish.

INGREDIENTS

vegetables (your choice from the *All You Can Eat Vegetable Buffet*)

½ head cauliflower, cored and separated into florets

¾ cup mushrooms, sliced

1 teaspoon salt

1 teaspoon black pepper

½ avocado

¾ cup coconut milk

2 cloves garlic

SUPPLIES

measuring cups and spoons

sharp knife

medium pot

food processor

medium oven-safe dish

Preheat the oven to 425°F.

Bring water to a boil in a pot and cook the vegetables of your choice.

Place the cauliflower into a food processor.

Blend until the cauliflower looks like large pieces of rice.

In a medium oven-safe dish, add the cauliflower, mushrooms, salt, and pepper.

In a food processor, blend the avocado, coconut milk, and garlic.

Combine the mixtures and place the dish in the oven for about 25 minutes, stirring occasionally.

Plate alongside your choice of vegetables and enjoy hot.

Snacks

Cranberry Zest Power Bars

You might have had the chance to experiment with power bars if you selected them as part of your snacks during the past three weeks. If not, don't worry—these are simple and fast to make. This variation of the Power Bar recipe is packed with flavor, antioxidants, and vitamin C.

INGREDIENTS

1¼ cups walnuts

1 cup dried cranberries

grated zest of 1 orange

⅓ cup egg white protein powder (optional)

2 tablespoons water

2 tablespoons freshly squeezed orange juice

SUPPLIES

measuring cups

food processor

large glass dish

Place the walnuts in a food processor and pulse for about 20 seconds, or until granular.

Add the cranberries, orange zest, protein powder, water, and orange juice and pulse for about 45 seconds, or until thoroughly combined.

Scoop the mixture into a square or rectangular dish and press down firmly. An 8x8-inch dish makes 10 to 12, half-inch-thick power bars.

Cut the pressed mixture into squares of your desired serving size and place the dish in the refrigerator to set for about an hour.

Serve once cooled or keep refrigerated and snack on these bars throughout the week.

Jalapeño Cauliflower Hummus

You're probably familiar with our hummus recipes by now. This week we're going to spice it up a little bit by adding roasted jalapeños! If you're not crazy about spice, feel free to substitute a different flavor or just use one of the past weeks' recipes.

INGREDIENTS

1 jalapeño, cut in half and seeded

1 head of cauliflower, cored and cut into quarter-size florets

2 tablespoons cumin powder

1½ tablespoons coconut oil, melted

4 cloves garlic, halved

½ cup tahini

2 lemons, squeezed

¼ cup water

¼ cup olive oil

5 carrots, for dipping

SUPPLIES

measuring cups and spoons

sharp knife

large mixing bowl

medium oven-safe dish

food processor

Preheat the oven to 450°F.

Place the jalapeño cut-side down on the oven rack and roast until the skin starts to blister and turn black. This should begin to happen about 10 minutes in.

Remove the jalapeño from the oven and allow to cool.

In a large mixing bowl, mix the cauliflower florets, cumin, coconut oil, and garlic (you may want to use your hands).

Pour the mixture into a baking dish and place in the oven to bake for about 30 minutes, or until the cauliflower turns a light golden brown.

Remove from the oven and let cool for 10 minutes.

Place the cauliflower mixture into a food processor.

Add the jalapeño, tahini, lemon juice, and water, and blend until smooth.

Scrape the sides of the processor to ensure the mixture blends thoroughly.

Stream in the olive oil and pulse for about a minute.

Serve warm or refrigerate and serve chilled within four days.

Use carrots for dipping.

TIP: For a less garlicky version, replace the fresh garlic with garlic powder. This is recommended if you plan to enjoy the hummus over a couple of days.

Spicy Jerky

Continuing with this week's spice theme, this jalapeño jerky snack is based on the basic recipe we've been using throughout the Cleanse, with the simple addition of a little spice.

INGREDIENTS

1 (4- to 5-pound) frozen beef roast

1 (8- to 10-ounce) bottle balsamic vinegar

1 (8-ounce) bottle coconut aminos

1 jalapeño, diced small

2 tablespoons red pepper flakes

1 teaspoon salt

½ cup honey

SUPPLIES

measuring cups

sharp knife

marinade bowl

aluminum foil

baking sheet

Place the frozen roast out to defrost until the outside rim of the roast is soft but the center is still frozen.

Slice the roast into strips that are about ⅛-inch thick and place the strips in a bowl.

Pour a 50:50 ratio of balsamic vinegar and coconut aminos into the bowl to almost cover the beef strips.

Add in the diced jalapeño, red pepper flakes, salt, and honey, and stir until the marinade coats all the beef.

Allow the mixture to sit and marinate for at least 2 hours (overnight in the refrigerator is better if time allows).

Preheat the oven to 190°F.

Place the beef strips onto a foil-lined baking sheet.

Place in the oven to bake and flip about every 30 minutes.

To test if the jerky is done, fold a piece in half and look for white threads. If you see the white threads, it's finished cooking.

Once done, remove the jerky from the oven and allow to cool before serving; or refrigerate and enjoy within five days.

TIP: Make sure you cut the jerky thin enough; otherwise you'll get little, not-so-tasty steaks. Also, having the meat slightly frozen will make it easier to cut. Use a serrated knife and keep hot water running to run your hands under—they will get cold!

Berries or Fruit, Dried Dates, Raw Nuts, and All You Can Eat Vegetable Buffet

These snack staples remain consistent from the previous weeks. Please visit Chapter 12 and 13 to review information about these great snack choices.

Week Four: The Home Stretch!

You've selected your *Meal Plan* and you're fired up because this is your last full week on the Cleanse! Stay strong this week as you complete your Cleanse journey. As you wrap up, remember to take some time to review your accomplishments and tips. It's easy to get a little too relaxed as you draw near to the end of your journey, so stay focused this week, and if you start to waver, think back on all that you've accomplished so far. You'll also want to begin thinking about where you'd like to go from here, and if you might like to continue your journey into a full-time Paleo lifestyle. We'll provide more information to help you make this decision in Chapter 17, so stay tuned!

Week Four Tips
Learn What You Like

You've spent a lot of time over the last few weeks eating Paleo-friendly foods and in the process have no doubt determined what you like and what you don't enjoy. We encourage you to take some time and look back on this. Getting to know your preferences will help prolong your healthy eating habits.

Pay Attention to the Transformation

Undoubtedly your body has experienced a great deal of change since you set out on your Paleo Cleanse journey. You've probably noticed physical changes, such as slimming down, skin clarity, and a more toned appearance, as well as other welcome changes, such as steady blood sugar levels and increased energy. Acknowledge the changes you are seeing and feeling. Reflecting upon your past weeks and understanding how the Paleo Cleanse has affected you in a positive manner will keep you motivated to stay committed to the end.

Eat Often and Drink Water Regularly

Staying hydrated and eating regularly are two simple things that can make a huge difference and will help you stay on track during your last week.

An interesting note is that the body often reacts the same way to being thirsty as it does to being hungry. If you're dehydrated, your body can send signals to your mind that lead you to believe that you're hungry. Prevent yourself from cheating or overeating in these instances by taking care of your most basic need—hydration.

Habits Have Formed…Don't Break Them

The end of Week Three (Day 21) was the turning point. Now, in your fourth week of Paleo commitment, you are beginning to solidify new, healthy habits to replace your pre-Cleanse lifestyle. Your old, potentially unhealthy habits are being rewritten with habits that support your future. Stay committed to your routine this week, as this will assist you both in completing the Cleanse and in the choices you make thereafter.

Plan Your Meals

Having premade meals and planning ahead of time is a surefire way to increase your chances of success. Not planning ahead, not shopping in advance, and not sticking to cooking days (at the very least to prepare your snacks) greatly increases your chance of cheating. You're in your last week now—don't allow yourself the chance to cheat. Be prepared, premake your Paleo meals, and ensure that you have ample Paleo snacks on hand. Plan ahead and finish strong!

Your Taste Buds Are Changing

One of the things that we noticed during Week Four was that our taste buds began to change. We preferred fresh fruits, vegetables, and protein over pre-Cleanse foods like bread, oatmeal, and pasta. You'll no doubt begin to notice this change as well; and, the longer you choose to stay on the Paleo Diet, the more noticeable this change will become for you. Embrace the change—it's a healthy one—and it's your body's way of righting itself to eat what is healthy and what sustains it.

You may still have some cravings now and then (which is normal); after all you have probably been eating those foods for many years and you're not going to kill all of your cravings in a month alone. Just remember that experiencing regular cravings now is likely a mental thing, which means you have complete control over stopping them with the help of your new best friend—willpower. We know from personal experience that if you cheat, your cravings will only become worse, so if you feel like you need something badly or that your willpower needs a check-in, take a look back at Chapter 11's Learn to Fight Cravings.

You're Comfortable, Enjoy It

You're probably getting comfortable at this point in your Cleanse. You're starting to truly feel the benefits of healthy eating, you understand the impact that food choices have on your life and you have a good idea of what Paleo-friendly foods you enjoy, as well as how to make them. Enjoy this point in the process. Embrace the Paleo Cleanse as it becomes a new normality for you. The habits you are building this week will only add to your sense of comfort, so continue to focus on a healthy life and enjoy the comfort it brings.

Week Four Summary

Can you believe it?! You've made it through your last full week of the Paleo Cleanse! We want to take this time to congratulate you on all the hard work you've put into your personal Cleanse journey. Just remember to stay strong for the next two days.

Coming ahead, with the help of Part 4, you'll determine where the road to health leads you from here. You're always more likely to be successful if you have a plan. So make a plan for healthy living moving forward. In Part 5, we'll provide great resources for transitioning into the Paleo lifestyle full time. There are also numerous other resources located online at ThePaleoPact.com and in the *Recommended Reading* list in the back of this book. Even if you decide not to continue the Paleo Diet full-time, you may well enjoy a number of the recipes included in Chapter 22 and 23. Take a look, try them out, and let us know how you enjoy them; but first, focus on your final two Days of the Paleo Cleanse.

- You're almost done—keep going. You officially have two Days left of your Cleanse. Go out on a strong note!

- Take the time to determine what foods and recipes you like; understanding your preferences will keep you eating healthily.

- Pay attention to your transformation; don't get so caught up in the day-to-day that you don't see the overall benefits you are receiving from the Cleanse.

- The basics are critical to success; stay hydrated and eat regularly!

- Habits have formed. Don't break them. The best way to keep yourself from cheating is to plan your meals in advance.

- Your taste buds are changing. Don't be surprised if you start to like new foods, or if you suddenly dislike foods that you used to eat all the time.

- You've kicked your cravings, and that should mean that you're far more comfortable than when you started the Cleanse. Stay comfortable and don't give in to temptations.

CHAPTER 16

Paleo Cleanse, Week Five

Week Five, Yes That's Right!

The final two days are here. We're leaving their planning up to you—we know you've got this covered. Feel free to look back at all of the *Meal Plan* choices that we provided over the last four weeks and then create your custom *Meal Plan* for the final days. Go!

PERSONAL MEAL PLAN SELECTION

	BREAKFAST	SNACK	LUNCH	SNACK	DINNER
MONDAY					
TUESDAY					

The Paleo Cleanse Wrap-Up

Ummm...so what am I supposed to do next? This is that critical point where you have to decide how to move forward. Do you still want to keep following a Paleo lifestyle? We hope so, but maybe you have decided that you need to follow the Paleo Diet at large and make slight personal variations.

Living a Paleo lifestyle means eating foods that our human species is naturally designed to digest and living a well-balanced, active lifestyle. Are you going to lose all the good you've acquired while being strictly Paleo for one month if you have a cheat meal once in a while or even once a week? No. It is important to remember, though, that cheat foods can affect your body and create the vicious cycle of cravings. Our best advice to you is to listen to your body.

First, refer back to the *Pre-Cleanse and Post-Cleanse Checklists* from Chapter 5. You completed one worksheet before beginning the Paleo Cleanse. Those answers captured how you felt before you began your journey to health. Take a few minutes to fill out your "after" chart and then compare it to your original chart. What changes are you seeing with your body? Did you lose weight or body fat? Or maybe you've gotten rid of those horrible headaches you used to get. Perhaps the difference is as vague as simply feeling better.

We recommend using these worksheets as a guide to your body. Think about what they tell you about this 30-day dietary change and how continuing to nourish and support your body can protect your future health. Whatever your personal results are, be proud of your accomplishment. Remember that the physical changes are miniscule compared to the health changes within each cell of your body.

The Paleo Cleanse Is Over, Why Am I Still Reading?

The next section of the book was added to provide you with tips and resources to continue your Paleo journey if you would like to do so. We hope you do! You will find details about foods that were restricted on the Cleanse, but which you can now happily introduce into your diet, as well as more information about the various schools of Paleo and the more modern thoughts on dairy.

We will also discuss the most common criticisms of the Paleo Diet and why the Paleo community, backed by research and medical doctors, don't believe these concerns to be valid.

We go on to share a number of the most frequently asked questions we encountered and how best to answer them. We also provide you with a chapter dedicated to Paleo alternatives to things like soda and pasta, which you may think you couldn't possibly live without long-term. But before we go into detail on any of that, we promised you we'd have a celebratory dessert recipe waiting, so without further ado, here it is!

Decadent Chocolate Chip Cookies

INGREDIENTS

1 cup tapioca flour

¼ cup coconut flour

¼ teaspoon baking soda

½ teaspoon salt

½ cup grass-fed butter

½ cup coconut palm sugar

5 teaspoons water

½ cup dark chocolate chips

arrowroot flour, as a nonstick base for rolling

SUPPLIES

measuring cups and spoons

aluminum foil or parchment paper

large baking sheet

small mixing bowl

food processor

rolling pin

cookie cutter

Preheat the oven to 325°F.

Place foil or parchment paper sheets over your baking sheet.

Combine the tapioca flour, coconut flour, baking soda, and salt in a small bowl.

In a food processor, pulse the butter and sugar for about 2 minutes, or until fluffy.

Add the dry ingredients and water to the butter and sugar mixture and pulse until well combined.

Fold the chocolate chips into the cookie mixture.

Lightly dust arrowroot flour on a clean counter.

Using a rolling pin, roll the cookie dough until ¼-inch thick and then cut out your cookies using a cookie cutter.

Place the cut cookies on your lined baking sheet and bake for 12 to 14 minutes.

Remove from the oven and allow to cool for about 10 minutes before serving.

We picked chocolate chip cookies as the celebratory dessert because they are such a traditional and well-liked treat. That said, if you prefer other desserts like brownies, date balls, or citrus Popsicles, we have plenty of other dessert options available for you in Chapter 23. Pick your favorite, get baking—truly enjoy it (with a lavish almond milk latte or a glass of champagne!)—and then return to journey with us beyond the Cleanse.

PART 4

DAY 31 AND BEYOND

CHAPTER 17

Living Paleo

At this point you may be dabbling with the idea of continuing a Paleo lifestyle, or you may already have decided that after the amazing transformations, you simply cannot live any other way. Whatever stage you are at, the overview below, including various Paleo schools of thought and post-Cleanse guidelines, will help you choose food wisely.

Varying Schools of Thought

The Paleolithic Era can be thought of as the original school of Paleo. We delved into this in the very first chapter, so to avoid repetition we'll summarize this school as follows: living entirely off the earth and from the gain of hunting. Our ancestors ate what gave them the energy to hunt and gather and avoided that which didn't (grains and legumes). There was no baking, no dairy, and no refined sugar.

The earliest modern school of Paleo is the one popularized by Loren Cordain. This version closely resembles the original school of Paleo and may therefore be considered fairly strict. This school does not promote the consumption of Paleo desserts (due to sugar and flour quantities, although technically Paleo), is strongly against any dairy consumption (with the sole exception of butter, a recent addition), does not advocate honey or agave nectar, remains against the intake of white potatoes, and does not promote the notion of bacon as a Paleo-friendly food.

The newer schools of Paleo are a little more lenient because they recognize that people have different heritages and are therefore accustomed to different food types. For example, Asians have been eating a diet largely based on white rice for decades, without any notable health effects. Similarly, descendants of European countries have been enjoying dairy for far longer than many countries in Africa, for example. The people of Europe are therefore more likely to be lactase persistent.[33] This more contemporary school of thought subsequently encourages people to begin with a strict detox to return the body to its normal state—this you have already completed with your 30-Day Paleo Cleanse—and then to slowly introduce foods like grass-fed milk and cheese into your diet and see how your body reacts. This newer version of the Paleo lifestyle is commonly referred to as the Primal Diet.

There are some members of this contemporary, Primal school who feel white potatoes are okay to consume, while others still disagree with this (we personally restrict our intake of white potatoes). The same applies to Paleo desserts. Many Primal supporters feel that all desserts should be restricted, while others feel that because the ingredients are Paleo, you can happily consume them without portion control. One thing that this contemporary school all tends to agree on is that bacon is a perfectly acceptable part of one's diet (we wouldn't have it any other way!) and that dark chocolate (typically above 85 percent cacao) is not harmful, either.

To help you decide where you best fit in with the varying schools of thought and degrees of stringency, we begin by reviewing post-Cleanse Paleo food groups for long-term consumption.

Post-Cleanse Paleo Lifestyle

During the Paleo Cleanse we suggested limiting your intake of a number of foods that are actually considered Paleo, such as healthy starches and sugary fruits. We recommended this because, while these foods are Paleo and perfectly natural, they still dispense a large amount of glucose into the body. Consequently, in order to detox quickly and experience results in just 30 days, these foods were strategically reduced. Now that your Cleanse is complete, these foods are all freely available to you.

Let's look at the full list of foods to favor and those to avoid when living a Paleo lifestyle. It should help you pinpoint how to proceed from here.

Paleo-Unfriendly Foods	Notes
Refined Sugar	Continue to avoid
Industrial Foods	Continue to avoid
Gluten	Avoid at all costs
Grains	Continue to avoid; if you do cheat, cheat with white rice
Dairy	Continue to avoid, except for grass-fed butter; introduce grass-fed milk and cheese slowly if desired
Legumes	Continue to avoid
Vegetable Oils	Avoid at all costs
Soda	Avoid at all costs; refer to the substitute section later in this chapter
Candy	Avoid at all costs
Chips	Continue to avoid, or substitute with sweet potato chips made with coconut oil
Pasta	Continue to avoid; refer to the substitute section later in this chapter

Cleanse-Eliminated Paleo Foods	Notes
All Paleo Flours	Enjoy in moderation
Coconut Palm Sugar	Enjoy in moderation
Date Sugar	Enjoy in moderation
Grass-fed Butter	Enjoy in moderation
Alcohol	Enjoy in moderation; stick to gluten-free alcohol and wine
Fruit Juice/Juicing	Continue to avoid store-bought fruit juice; blend, don't juice (you lose the fiber juicing)

Cleanse-Restricted Paleo Foods	Notes
Nuts	Enjoy happily; keep your intake moderate if you are trying to lose weight
Natural Fats	Enjoy happily
Healthy Starches	Enjoy happily; keep your intake moderate if you are trying to lose weight
Natural Sweeteners	Enjoy in moderation
Sugary Fruits	Enjoy happily; keep your intake moderate if you are trying to lose weight or notice any blood sugar spikes

Cleanse-Approved Paleo Foods	Notes
Vegetables	Enjoy happily; continue to eat as much as you like
Leafy Greens	Enjoy happily; continue to eat as much as you like
Meats	Enjoy happily, including the fat
Fish	Enjoy happily, stick to wild-caught (captive-raised are not always fed their natural diet)
Eggs	Enjoy happily, with the yolks
Low-Sugar Fruits	Enjoy happily; keep your intake moderate if you are trying to lose weight or notice any blood sugar spikes
Unsweetened Tea	Enjoy happily
Coffee	Enjoy happily with Paleo-friendly sweeteners and creamers
Water, coconut water	Enjoy happily (room temperature is most easily absorbed by your body), hydrate often

Now that you have a clear guide to each food group through the eyes of the Paleo Diet, you can decide how strict you wish to be and if you would like to introduce any foods accepted by the contemporary school.

The Art of Introducing Foods

If you do decide to align with the contemporary school of Paleo and wish to see if you can introduce some foods into your diet, do it very slowly. Introduce one thing at a time, beginning with a very small quantity. Continue this for a couple of days and see how you feel. Be on the lookout for changes in your blood sugar, sleeping habits, energy levels, skin clarity, headaches, or stomach complications. Ensure you know whether you can or cannot tolerate the food product before trying to introduce another food item.

Please note that while the consumption of certain foods may not have an immediate effect on your body, there remain a number of food groups that have been scientifically proven to negatively affect your body in the long-term. These include the all-time no-no's: grains, legumes, vegetable oils, and refined sugar. Cut those out full-time if you can. Introductory items, such as grass-fed dairy, should never be consumed in large quantities, regardless if you are lactase persistent or not. The same applies to Paleo flours and fruit sugars (such as coconut palm sugar and date sugar). Enjoy these items in desserts once in a while refrain from letting them become a staple part of your diet—they are sugar after all.

Getting Friendly with Fats

No matter what school of Paleo you choose to align with, the consensus on the natural fat found in animal protein remains the same—it's good for you.[34] Yes, we are well aware that fat has been made to look like a demon and gnawing into a fatty strip on the edge of your sirloin steak takes guts. The thing is, fat played a large role in developing our species into the intelligent human beings we are today.

Repeat after us: I am not afraid of fat! In all seriousness, and to put your mind even more at ease, fat is even less concerning when you are consuming meat from animals that have been grass fed. Why does grass-fed make a difference? Firstly, studies have shown that grass-fed meat is lower in total fat, has a healthier ratio of omega-3 to omega-6 fatty acids, and is lower in saturated fat.[35] Secondly, fat is like a sponge. Grass-fed meat comes from animals that have been fed their natural diet, so the fat absorbs nothing unnatural, unlike meat from animals that have been fed grain-based, vegetarian, hormone-induced diets that have been treated with pesticides.

Plus, remember when we examined the traditional Food Pyramid in Chapter 2? *MyPyramid* and *MyPlate* suggest that carbohydrates and vegetables, rather than fats and vegetables, should account for our primary caloric intake. John Durant points out in his book *The Paleo Manifesto* that "grains—the base of the USDA Food Pyramid for humans—are what American farmers use to fatten up their livestock."[36] It's not fat that you have to worry about.

What about Foods I Can't Live Without?

We understand that you have probably enjoyed certain Paleo-unfriendly foods much of your life and can't possible imagine living without them. That's okay, we have those "can't live without" food items, too, and we also have Paleo-friendly solutions!

In Chapter 22 you will find recipes that provide easy alternatives to those common foods and drinks that most people simply cannot imagine living without long-term. With those great alternatives, there are even fewer excuses to discontinue your journey to health.

What about What Others Think?

You mean, until they notice how amazing you look and want to know where you got your hands on this book?! Kidding aside, we know that it's hard to go against the status quo, and this diet certainly contradicts just about everything we've been taught about health. Yet, it's *the* original, oldest, and longest diet our species has ever followed.

The chapter ahead covers the best advice we have for sharing your Paleo discoveries with the curious and answering the questions of the critics.

CHAPTER 18

Curiosity and Criticism

Paleo is popular, and with good reason. However, when something is in the spotlight, it attracts attention, both good and bad. While we would like to believe that most people understand the concept of eating clean (avoiding industrial, modified foods), there are and always will be the outspoken NBs: the Non-Believers. That's okay. We are big advocates of doing what is best for one's own body, within reason, of course. We are here to help you, not only with Paleo shopping lists and recipes, but also with frequently asked questions and answers (coming up in Chapter 19) so you can confidently explain your case to the NBs.

To give you an idea of some of the criticism surrounding the Paleo Diet, we delve into a few misconceptions below.

In the 2013 *U.S. News & World Report* ranking of "Best Diets," the Paleo Diet tied with the high-protein, low-carb Dukan Diet in last place. Saving the best for last? We think so! In all seriousness, why did the Paleo Diet rank so low? First, the critics said it was too hard to replicate an Ancestral diet in our modern times; second, they said it eliminated food groups that were necessary for vital nutrients; and third, they said that to pull it off would be too pricey.

We've solved the first and third "problems" by walking you through easy-to-make recipes and tasty snack ideas, so following a Paleo Diet will never be an issue, and we'll share all the best places to find essential Paleo ingredients at the best possible prices. The second "problem" makes little sense when you consider our natural human diet. Yes, the Paleo Diet does eliminate food groups—grains, dairy, and legumes—but because the human body was not designed to digest nutrients from those food groups anyway, they serve little purpose and the concern becomes invalid. Plus, these nutrients are easily gained (and in higher quantities) from other Paleo-friendly food groups.

Finally, the Paleo Diet is sometimes referred to as a "fad diet" comparable to the Atkins Diet. The funny thing about that is that this diet has been around for longer than any other. It's *the* diet our ancestors followed. It's *the* diet that enabled us to develop into a highly intelligent species. It's the *only* diet that's 2.6 million years old. So, as C. J. Hunt quotes Dr. Boyd Eaton in the final words of his documentary *The Perfect Human Diet*, "If this is a fad diet, it's a 2 million year old fad."

Common Concerns

Some of the most common concerns and criticisms that surface when discussing the Paleo Diet often stem from subjects such as: the life span of our ancestors; the belief that whole grains are essential to the human diet; the relationship between calcium and dairy; the fear of cholesterol in high-protein, high-fat diets; and the push toward vegetarianism. Let's briefly discuss each of these apprehensions so that you feel confident in your newfound direction and know how to address these common questions with others.

Ancestral Life Span: When discussing the Paleo Diet, it's very common for the discussion regarding the life span of our ancestors to arise. The question normally posed is: Why would we choose to live a Paleo lifestyle when our Paleolithic ancestors only lived to about 40 years of age? There are two things to consider when discussing this topic: evidence and lifestyle.

The fact is, we have little evidence confirming how long our ancestors actually lived. Due to natural, unassisted birth and the lack of modern-day medication, our ancestors experienced an unfortunate number of child deaths. This significantly decreases the average life expectancy data we are presented with.

The second point to discuss is lifestyle. It's very difficult to draw a fair comparison between the life span of our ancestors and our own when the lifestyle we live is completely different. Back then, the wilderness, the seasons, and the elements all played a role, along with predators. Advances in medicine that greatly increase life expectancy today, such as operations, hospitals, and life-support systems, did not exist. What we do know from skeletal studies, however, is that our ancestors had strong bones, developing brains, healthy bodies, and perfect teeth.[37]

The Theory of Adaptation: We've come a long way since the Paleolithic Era. We certainly don't live the same lifestyle any longer and we haven't in quite some time. Consequently, the question, "Haven't we evolved to eat contemporary food products by now?" is often raised. The answer is no. The evidence is all around us with alarming (and climbing) obesity statistics and disease rates. We have evolved as beings, but our digestive tracts and the way we consume foods has not. We also have to remember that in the grand scheme of things, the time frame in which contemporary foods and agricultural by-products have been available to us is miniscule in the history of our species. A few thousand years is not a long enough time for any significant changes as a result of evolution to take place. Perhaps in time we will adapt to eat high-carbohydrate, high-sugar foods, but until then, we will continue to pay the price if we don't restrict them.

The Belief in Whole Grains: Whole grains are supposed to be healthy, aren't they? The push toward whole grains has gained traction over the past few years; suddenly, everyone thinks that consuming large quantities of oats, whole wheat breads, and brown rice is essential to our human diet. We understand the concept—whole grains sound a whole lot better for you than refined grains—but evolutionary science shows us that our ancestors didn't eat grains at all (and for good reason).

We've covered the dirty details about grain in previous chapters and uncovered the truth about their toxic protein tricks to ensure they remain intact in order to propagate as nature intended. We also learned that refined grains such as white rice are actually the healthier option (even though they technically have less nutritional content). This is because during the refinement process, much of the toxic proteins are stripped from the bran, enabling us to absorb more nutrients.

We think you've got this one down by now, but just in case you need a little refresher, you might want to revisit Chapter 3's discussion about whole and refined grains.

The Concern about Calcium: The concern over not getting enough calcium to ensure we have strong bones has been fostered over the past century by dairy industry marketing. Do we really need to supplement calcium? And can we get calcium from other, healthier sources? The answer is no to the first question and yes to the second.

Studies have shown that the hyped concern over getting enough calcium to ensure our bones are strong enough to withstand old age has led to numerous other health issues. Various studies have blamed excess calcium for an increased risk of heart attacks, kidney stones, bowel disorders, and strokes.[38] Since there is already calcium naturally found in many of the foods we consume (especially foods advocated by the Paleo Diet), we really don't need to be concerned about not getting enough.

Luckily, other studies focused on bone health have come to the conclusion that continual force (from exercise), along with vitamin D, vitamin K2, and magnesium citrate (naturally found in foods) are more effective in preserving bone density. So, ditch the milk and eat your vegetables!

The Cholesterol Myth: You know what we're referring to—the ingrained belief that high-fat and high-protein diets, like the Paleo Diet, increase cholesterol and the likelihood of cardiovascular disease. It's a fear that's been cultivated in our society over the past few decades, yet research and numerous doctors around the globe continue to point out that there is in fact no solid evidence that correlates high-fat and high-protein diets with high cholesterol or with cardiovascular disease. In fact, diets such as the Paleo Diet have shown to decrease body weight, body mass index, blood pressure, and plasma insulin. These are all factors that reduce the risk of cardiovascular disease. On the contrary, low-fat and high-carbohydrate diets (typical of our contemporary Western diet) have caused an influx in body weight and heart-related diseases. So the next time you crack an egg, savor the yolk and release your fear of the unsubstantiated cholesterol myth.[39]

Vegetarianism/Veganism: The idea of consuming animal protein has been under scrutiny a lot lately. Vegetarianism and veganism are growing philosophies across the globe, arguing two main concerns: that eating meat is both cruel and unhealthy. Let's address each of these viewpoints.

Regarding the first vegetarianism concern over meat consumption, we absolutely agree that eating meat can be cruel—those animals kept in tiny indoor pens, being fed grains and injected with hormones to make them grow as big as possible as quickly as possible do not live happy lives. We're not against their thoughts on this at all; in fact, we align with them. But animals living on natural pastures eating their natural diet of grass and being well cared for have an entirely different life experience. Yes, they still go to the butcher—the food chain continues to exist—but the cruelty factor becomes far less of an issue.

The second stance vegetarianism takes about meat being unhealthy doesn't truthfully make sense when you think about the scientific evolution of our species. If you ask an evolutionary biologist if they think any of our ancestors were vegetarian, they tend to laugh and shake their heads, as we saw in the documentary *The Perfect Human Diet.* According to evolutionary biology, it was animal protein and animal fats that enabled our bodies and brains to develop and advance beyond our fellow creatures in the wilderness into the intelligent species we are today. Moreover, the idea that adequate sources of protein can be gained from a vegetarian diet is highly questioned within the Paleo community. In order to get protein from non-animal sources, vegetarians typically turn to soy, which is part of the legume family. As you know from earlier discussions in the book, legumes are problematic to the human digestive system and can cause intestinal inflammation, resulting in autoimmune disruption and various diseases.

Last, we have also heard the argument that research on vegetarianism has been around longer than research on the Paleo Diet. That's certainly debatable. Vegetarianism was popularized in the mid-1800s, while the Paleo Diet was first popularized a decade earlier, in the mid-1700s. The fact also remains that the Ancestral diet has been around since the very beginning of our species (2.6 million years ago), while the earliest records of vegetarianism cited are from the fifth century BCE—that's too many years difference to calculate!

Now that we've reviewed the most common reservations about the Paleo Diet and looked briefly into the research-based reasons why the Paleo community doesn't believe these concerns to be valid, let's take a look at some basic questions that will no doubt be asked of you and ideas on how best to respond to them.

CHAPTER 19

FAQ and Paleo Answers

You know the research is grounded in science, but the majority of the population does not (and the Non-Believers don't want to believe it). So, they're calling you Fred and Wilma Flintstone, they tease you (hopefully in good nature) about eating rabbit food, and picture you hunting for your meat on a daily basis with a spear in one hand and a loincloth around your now leaner Paleo body? We're not exaggerating! Believe us, we've heard it all at this point.

How should you react? Smile and tell them that is exactly right. Why not go even further and say that you're exhausted after the hunt but the 20 pounds of fresh meat was really worth it! Trust us on this one—going along with the mockery never fails to stop these types of insinuations, so just have fun with it.

We've collected a little ensemble of Paleo humor that we house on ThePaleoPact.com. You can even show your critics the fantastic memes, videos, and quotes on the subject. Humor is a great way to break down the critique barrier. As always, we encourage you to share your own stories and humor; unity is where we get our strength in the Paleo community. Unity and the several hours we put in each day lifting boulders and hunting mammoths. Just kidding!

Plus, as you continue to feel better, gain energy, improve your skin tone, and drop those unwanted pounds, you will be the last one laughing. Enjoy it!

Below are a few common questions and examples of how we respond to them. We hadn't expected these questions when we started the Cleanse, but by the end of Week Four we were pros at answering them!

Ohhh...so you only eat raw food?

No. While the Paleo Diet is centered around the consumption of natural foods, we, as our cavemen did, have mastered cookery.

So you have to kill food with your bare hands right? (We wish we were joking about this one.)

No. Luckily I can get my food at the grocery store, just like you.

Isn't that one of those diets where you don't eat anything?

Actually I get to eat a lot. In fact, I can eat way more than I used to because the food I eat now is more easily absorbed by the body and has fewer calories. Jealous!?

Why would you want to eat like a caveman? I mean they barely made it past 40.

It's true that our life spans are much longer now, but that's largely due to modern medicine and the fact that we are not exposed to the wild situations that our ancestors were. Cavemen had excellent teeth, toned bodies, and active lifestyles. That's what we're going for.

But whole grains are healthy—why would you eliminate them?

Technically, yes, they have healthy nutrients. The thing is, the human body cannot absorb those nutrients because they are trapped inside a layer of toxic proteins. Grains are made to propagate and to do so were designed to pass through the body. All we gain from consuming them is a feeling of being full, accompanied by an insulin high and intestinal inflammation, which have numerous detrimental health risks, like diabetes and obesity.

Wait, so you can't drink any alcohol?

Would we do this if we couldn't?! In most schools, the same Paleo principles apply to drinks, as they do for food. For example, we would avoid traditional beer because of the gluten. Wine and cider, however, are healthier alternatives (in small quantities, of course). There's also tequila—it's made from a plant!

You know we've progressed from our caveman days, right?

Yes, we do know that. Thanks to our ancestors' diet of animal protein and vegetables, we developed our large human brains, which have enabled us to progress culturally and technologically into the advanced species we are today. That said, our digestive systems have not changed. The natural foods we consumed then enabled us to get here, but ever since the boom of Agriculture our health has steadily declined. Our bodies are simply not adapted to eat the high doses of sugar, grains, and industrial foods that are common today. Also, just because we're living longer doesn't mean we're living healthier lives.

Everything in moderation! Isn't that a better way to eat than cutting out major food groups?

Okay, so you're saying we can eat a little bit of candy, with a little bit of soda, with a little bit of pizza, with a little bit of burger, with a little bit of grilled cheese, and that's healthy because it's all in moderation? The saying "everything in moderation" only applies if the majority of one's diet is healthy. Unfortunately, with our twenty-first century diets, most people do not eat healthily. Also, a lot of the nutrients that you find in food groups that are not considered Paleo can be found in (and more easily digested in the form of) fruits and vegetables.

———————— ⫘ ————————

If you have more questions, or you encounter more criticism of your new dietary direction, there's nothing wrong with admitting that you haven't yet learned a particular aspect and that you will find out the good reasoning behind it. Then simply send us a message via

ThePaleoPact.com and we'll provide the answer or research the answer for you. There is typically a large amount of biology and health-based research explaining each element of the Paleo philosophy because it is a dietary lifestyle founded on evolutionary science.

PART 5

MAKING PALEO
MANAGEABLE

CHAPTER 20

Allergy Substitutions

Allergies are a challenging thing and can unfortunately make it very hard to implement lifestyle changes or try a new diet or cleanse. Thankfully, the Paleo Diet is easy to navigate if you do have food allergies. Take it from our own experience: You can have a food allergy and find success with a Paleo lifestyle. Quite honestly, you may find it easier to do the Paleo Diet than your normal diet, simply because the Paleo Diet, and lifestyle in general, restrict several of the common food allergies.

In this section we will discuss some of the most common food allergies and their relation to the Paleo Diet. We'll also address how to substitute foods if you find that something you're allergic to is included in one of our recipes. We want to ensure that no matter what your dietary restrictions, you are successful on your Paleo journey.

The Common Food Allergens

While it is possible to be allergic to almost anything, there are eight common allergens that make up 90 percent of all food-based allergic reactions.[40]

These top-eight food allergens are:

- peanuts
- tree nuts

- milk
- eggs
- wheat
- soy
- fish
- shellfish

We're going to take a minute to discuss each of these food allergens and how they might impact your Paleo journey. We'll also provide substitutes for these foods where applicable.

Peanuts

This one is easy. Peanuts are considered a legume, and legumes are not a food group that's consumed on the Paleo Diet. There are various reasons for this. A large factor is that they exacerbate inflammation and they just didn't exist during the Paleolithic Era. We do not use peanut products in our recipes, so you don't need to concern yourself with any substitutions or exclusions for peanuts.

Tree Nuts

The tree nut group is generally composed of walnuts, almonds, hazelnuts, cashews, pistachios, and Brazil nuts. You may have an allergy to all of these, or perhaps just to one. Please be aware that many of our recipes do include tree nuts; they are a common ingredient in our recipes because they are dense and provide a good substitute for grains in things like protein bars.

Tree nuts are included in our recipes as (but not limited to):
- the actual nut
- almond milk
- flours (e.g., we use almond flour in some of our recipes)

The following is a list of substitutions that you can use in our recipes (if you know of others, please feel free to use your own Paleo-friendly substitutes):

- If you're not allergic to all tree nuts, substitute with a different tree nut.
- Coconut milk is a great substitute for almond milk.
- Arrowroot, coconut, or tapioca flours are great substitutes for almond flour.

Milk

Milk is another easy allergy to avoid as it's not consumed on the Paleo Diet. The human body was not developed to ingest dairy after the breast-feeding stage, and this is evident in the large number of people who have dairy allergies or are lactase non-persistent.[41]

If you're trying to make a Paleo-unfriendly recipe Paleo-friendly, we recommend using almond or coconut milk as a milk substitute. If you're looking for creamer for your coffee or you just want a glass of milk, these are both good options. Other than that, dairy is generally not included in our recipes; the rare exception is ghee butter or grass-fed butter, which you can substitute with olive oil or coconut oil (use coconut oil when possible in recipes that require heating of any kind, as olive oil has a high oxidization rate and becomes toxic when heated).

Eggs

Eggs can be a challenging thing to be allergic to; we know this mainly from Melissa's experience. While eggs can often be a staple of the Paleo Diet, you can still avoid them easily with some creative substitutions and by having ample recipes to choose from. That's why we provide you with both!

Our weekly *Meal Plans* offer several egg-free selections for breakfast that are high in protein. This way it is easy for you to avoid this allergy, especially during the morning hours when it can be difficult to find a recipe without an egg base. However, the following are some great options for egg substitutes when you are baking:

- Mix 1 tablespoon ground flaxseed and 3 tablespoons warm water. Let it stand for about 10 minutes until the water is absorbed. This is the equivalent of one egg.
- Mix ¼ cup applesauce (make sure it's Paleo-friendly) and 1 teaspoon of baking powder. This is also the equivalent of one egg.
- Mash ¼ cup banana. This also replaces one egg.
- Another thing you should consider is if you actually need the egg. You may need to practice, but sometimes, egg isn't really needed in recipes.

Wheat

Here we go again with the easy allergy avoidance. Wheat is not considered Paleo and is therefore not included in any of our recipes. Instead of wheat, we make breads and similar wheat-type foods using Paleo-friendly flours. We've spent a great deal of time coming up with Paleo versions of common wheat recipes, so even if you didn't do the Paleo Cleanse and only wanted to avoid wheat, you'd be excited about what we're offering. Take a look at Chapters 22 and 23 for some great wheat-free recipes for the things you love to eat. Pizza crust, anyone?

Soy

Soy, like peanuts, is a member of the legume family. As we discussed before, legumes are not a food group consumed on the Paleo Diet and are therefore not included in any of our recipes. You'll notice that we substitute soy sauce in our recipes with things such as coconut aminos, which provide the same great taste for items like teriyaki sauce, but are much healthier for us.

Fish

Fish is a healthy and lean way to get protein into your diet and is Paleo-friendly. Fish is included as an ingredient in some of our recipes; don't worry though, it is easily replaceable with other lean proteins.

If you're allergic to certain types of fish, try using the following substitutes:

- You can substitute another fish that you are not allergic to.
- You can substitute the fish for other lean proteins, including shellfish, chicken, turkey, bison, ostrich, lamb, or grass-fed beef.

Shellfish

Shellfish is another great way to get lean protein; however, it's not an option if you are allergic to it. As with fish, you can easily substitute this protein with another lean protein in our recipes.

If you're allergic to certain types of shellfish, try the following substitutes:

- You can substitute another shellfish that you are not allergic to.
- You can substitute the shellfish for other lean proteins, including fish, chicken, turkey, bison, ostrich, lamb, or grass-fed beef.

Everything Else

We discussed the eight most common food allergies, but they're not all of the food allergies out there. Don't stress about food allergies; they're actually pretty easy to accommodate on a Paleo Diet, especially since you'll be preparing the majority of the foods yourself. If you have another food allergy that we didn't discuss, simply experiment with replacing that ingredient with something similar that is also Paleo. For example, say you are allergic to honey, like Camilla is. No problem— simply try using raw agave nectar or coconut palm sugar. It may take a little time, but you'll find a substitute that works for you. We've also intentionally provided you with multiple *Meal Plan* options so that you can pick another recipe if needed.

Read Your Labels

While many of our ingredients are straightforward, it's good to know exactly what type of vegetable or protein you select. If you have a food allergy, you're probably already accustomed to reading labels and checking for allergens. That's great! If you don't typically do this, it's time to start, and here's a good example: Recently we tried sundried tomato bacon, only to find that it had soy and wheat in the flavoring.

We want to reinforce this practice of checking labels, especially since you'll be working with some new ingredients that you may not be used to. Not only will this help you avoid your food allergies, it will also help to ensure that you're eating strictly Paleo-friendly foods. Make sure you read your labels!

Always Go with Your Gut

If you have a food allergy, you know that at times you're just not comfortable with how a food is prepared. Maybe you're just getting paranoid it has something in it that might spur an allergic reaction. It's okay; we get this sometimes, too. Listen to yourself and your gut instincts. It's not worth getting sick over, especially when it is so easy to pick another meal or substitute an ingredient. Always listen to your body.

CHAPTER 21

Guide to Eating Out

Choose Well

For those times when you're on the go or feel like a break from your kitchen, we recommend the following restaurant food choices:

- salads (dressing-free, or with olive oil and balsamic vinegar)
- vegetables
- grilled fish
- grilled chicken
- sushi (without rice, unless you are Primal); no soy sauce or wasabi (unless it's real wasabi rather than dyed horseradish)
- steak
- lettuce wraps
- burgers without the bun
- fajitas without the tortilla shell
- seafood or raw bar (mussels, clams, oysters, etc.)
- vegetable broth soups

Avoid at All Costs

- vegetable oils
- breaded foods
- deep-fried foods
- processed foods
- fast foods
- flavored coffees

CHAPTER 22

Can't-Live-Without Recipes

There are some foods that you just can't live without. Don't worry, we understand and are here to help you out with the following recipes for those must-have items. We've converted the traditional recipes into easy-to-make Paleo-friendly versions.

We hope you enjoy these recipes thoroughly and rejoice in knowing that they are Paleo-friendly. If you don't see a recipe here that you were hoping for, visit ThePaleoPact.com; we update the site regularly with delicious recipes to ensure your Paleo adventure is an exciting one.

Paleo Pizza Crust

This is one of our personal favorites. To top it off, it's also egg-free, which can be a difficult thing to accomplish when you're baking without traditional ingredients. Enjoy!

INGREDIENTS

1 tablespoon ground flaxseed

½ cup + 3 tablespoons warm water

1 clove garlic, diced

1 cup tapioca flour

⅓ cup + 1 to 3 tablespoons coconut flour

1 teaspoon salt

1 teaspoon Italian seasoning

½ cup olive oil

SUPPLIES

measuring cups and spoons

1 small mixing bowl

2 medium mixing bowls

aluminum foil

pizza sheet

cutting board

rolling pin (optional)

Preheat the oven to 425°F.

Mix the flaxseed and 3 tablespoons water, then let it sit for about 10 minutes until the water is absorbed.

Add the garlic and ½ cup water to the bowl and set aside.

Mix the tapioca flour, ⅓ cup coconut flour, salt, and Italian seasoning in a small bowl until thoroughly combined.

Add the flaxseed mixture, garlic/water mixture, and olive oil to the dry ingredients. Combine until you get the consistency of thick mashed potatoes.

Add 1 tablespoon of coconut flour at a time and incorporate until the mixture becomes drier, like play dough.

Place a piece of foil over a pizza sheet.

On a cutting board, place the dough ball and begin to flatten it into a circular shape. Use a rolling pin if needed (you may want to dust in tapioca flour if the dough begins to stick), roll out the crust to be about ⅛-inch thick.

Place the pizza sheet foil side down on the crust, then flip the cutting board.

Slowly peel away the board so that only the crust is left on the foil.

Cook for 12 to 15 minutes until you reach your desired crispness. You can then cover with toppings, cooking for a few minutes longer until the toppings are warm.

Paleo Soda

Soda is something many people overindulge in. While it can taste fantastic, it is not good for you at all. The following is a great recipe for Paleo soda; it tastes like cream soda and is an excellent substitute if you ever get a soda craving.

INGREDIENTS

1 liter water

⅓ cup honey

SUPPLIES

SodaStream machine

Carbonate the water.

Add the honey and mix (you can adjust this amount to taste).

Enjoy!

Paleo Pudding

This is a dessert you don't need to feel bad about eating! Replace the cacao powder with vanilla or lime to vary this pudding.

INGREDIENTS

¾ cup coconut milk

3 tablespoons honey

¼ to ½ cup cacao powder (for a light chocolate taste use ¼ cup, for a rich chocolate taste use ½ cup)

1 tablespoon chia seeds

1 ripe avocado

SUPPLIES

measuring cups and spoons

sharp knife

food processor

Combine everything in a food processor and blend until smooth.

Place in the fridge for about 1 hour.

Serve chilled.

Paleo Bread

What can we say, there is just something about bread that is hard to give up. The following is a simple recipe for Paleo bread that you can pair with any of our recipes in this book.

INGREDIENTS

2 tablespoons coconut oil, divided

2 cups arrowroot flour

½ cup flax meal

¼ cup coconut flour

½ teaspoon baking soda

¼ teaspoon salt

5 eggs

1 tablespoon apple cider vinegar

1 tablespoon honey

SUPPLIES

measuring cups

food processor

8x5-inch bread pan

Preheat the oven to 350°F.

Grease a bread pan with 1 tablespoon coconut oil.

In a food processor, add all the dry ingredients and pulse for about 1 minute.

Add the eggs, other tablespoon of coconut oil, apple cider vinegar, and honey, and blend for about another minute.

Place in the oven to bake for about 35 minutes, or until a skewer poked through the center of the loaf comes out clean.

Remove from the oven and let cool before slicing.

Sweet Potato Brownies

Brownies may be the best things ever created, and we mean ever! Since this could potentially be a deal breaker for most people, we decided we needed to include a couple of Paleo options in this book (there's one in the *Bonus Recipes* chapter as well). Not only is this option Paleo, but it is also egg-free.

INGREDIENTS

2 tablespoons flaxseed

6 tablespoons warm water

2½ cups orange sweet potato, grated then chopped

3 teaspoons vanilla extract

½ cup melted honey

½ cup olive oil

1½ tablespoons baking soda

¾ cup cacao powder

3 tablespoons coconut flour

coconut oil, for greasing

SUPPLIES

measuring cups and spoons

grater

glass baking dish

Preheat the oven to 375°F.

In a large bowl, mix the flaxseed and warm water and let the mixture sit for about 10 minutes.

Add the sweet potato, vanilla, honey, olive oil, baking soda, and cacao powder to the bowl and mix.

Add the coconut flour to the bowl and mix for about another minute.

Scoop the mixture into a greased baking dish and press the mixture flat, so that it's about 1-inch high.

Cook for about 30 minutes. Remove from the oven and allow to cool before serving.

Paleo Pasta

Pasta is one of those quick-to-whip-up dishes that form a staple in many Western diets. Giving up pasta was a hard adjustment to make initially—and then we discovered almond flour pasta. Now we simply substitute almond flour pasta for wheat flour pasta whenever we're in the mood for an Italian dinner.

INGREDIENTS

almond flour pasta
(see the *Purchasing Directory* for a product recommendation)

pasta sauce

SUPPLIES

large pot

Bring water to a boil in a large pot and cook the pasta based on the product recommendation.

Refer to Chapter 23 to select a Paleo sauce option.

Wrap It Up

Coconut wraps are a great alternative to traditional flour wraps (you can also use lettuce as wraps). Coconut wraps are a little difficult to make, so we recommend purchasing them. See the *Purchasing Directory* for our favorite brand and places to purchase it.

Bonus Recipes

Kickstart Your Mornings

There's no need for artificial energy drinks when you can make healthy homemade boosts in no time at all. What's more, unlike the energy drinks on most grocery store shelves, these recipes provide natural energy that won't leave you crashing.

Aloe Cranberry Shot

Aloe vera juice is rich in amino acids, vitamins, and minerals. It alkalizes and detoxifies the body, aiding the digestive tract and boosting the immune system. It's a great way to help your body start the day!

INGREDIENTS

1 tablespoon aloe vera juice

1 ounce cranberry juice

SUPPLIES

measuring cup and spoon

shot glass

Pour the aloe vera juice into a shot glass.

Top up with cranberry juice.

Shoot it down!

Paleo Coffee Shot

Yes: Coffee is Paleo. It's the artificial creamer, refined sugar, and syrup flavors that make takeout coffee a bad idea. The coffee itself doesn't hurt.

INGREDIENTS

1 ounce brewed coffee

1 tablespoon coconut milk or almond milk

coconut sugar, to taste

SUPPLIES

measuring cup and spoon

shot glass or espresso cup

Pour the brewed coffee into the shot glass or espresso cup.

Add the coconut milk and sugar to taste.

Sip at your leisure while hot.

Orange Kombucha Shot

Kombucha is a probiotic beverage that supports the intestinal system and aids digestion. Drink up!

INGREDIENTS

1 ounce kombucha

½ orange, squeezed

SUPPLIES

measuring cup

shot glass

Pour the kombucha into the shot glass.

Top up with freshly squeezed orange juice.

Shoot or sip, as you prefer.

Chia Lime Shot

Chia seeds boast enormous quantities of fatty acids, which are more easily absorbed by the body when in liquid form. It's a South American secret that's been used as a natural energy drink for centuries.

INGREDIENTS

1 ounce water

½ tablespoon chia seeds

1 lime, squeezed

SUPPLIES

measuring cup and spoon

shot glass

Pour the water into the shot glass.

Add the chia seeds and stir.

Top up with freshly squeezed lime juice.

Let sit for 15 to 20 minutes, allowing for the chia seeds to expand in the liquid before drinking.

Lavish Lattes

Great news! You don't need to spend your money on takeout lattes when you can make better ones yourself. Enjoy these simple yet decadent liquid treats as you make your way to work, or savor in the afternoon as a delicious boost.

Iced Vanilla Latte

A delicious homemade iced latte free of refined sugar and artificial flavorings, this recipe also works well with almond milk if you prefer not to have the slight coconut flavor.

INGREDIENTS

ice

1 to 2 shots of brewed espresso

2 tablespoons honey

¼ teaspoon vanilla extract

¼ cup almond milk or coconut milk

SUPPLIES

measuring cup and spoons

coffee cup or to-go cup

Add ice to the cup.

Pour the espresso over the ice.

Add the honey and vanilla extract and stir.

Top with milk and enjoy.

Hot Vanilla Latte

This is the exact same recipe as the iced latte above, only this one is ice-free and served hot, for those colder days.

INGREDIENTS

1 to 2 shots of brewed espresso

2 tablespoons honey

¼ teaspoon vanilla extract

¼ cup almond milk or coconut milk

SUPPLIES

measuring cups

small sauté pan

coffee cup or to-go cup

Pour the espresso into the cup.

Add the honey and vanilla extract and stir.

In a small sauté pan, heat the milk over medium heat.

Pour the hot milk over the espresso and enjoy while warm.

Hot Green Tea Latte

This base recipe is the same as the one for the coffee lattes, substituting for antioxidant-rich green tea for the espresso.

INGREDIENTS

3 to 4 ounces of brewed green tea

2 tablespoons of honey

¼ teaspoon vanilla extract

¼ cup almond milk or coconut milk

SUPPLIES

measuring cups

small sauté pan

coffee cup or to-go cup

Pour the green tea into the cup.

Add the honey and vanilla extract and stir.

In a small sauté pan, heat the milk over medium heat.

Pour the hot milk over the tea and enjoy while warm.

Power Breakfasts

You know the drill: Breakfast is an important meal. It's old news and we're not going to dispute that, especially since on the Paleo Diet you can consume as many Paleo-friendly calories as you like. So indulge in protein-packed decadence to start your day enriched and you'll be ready for whatever life brings.

Apricot Almond Power Bars

Packed with the nutrients of apricots and almonds and powered with egg protein, these bars are a great midmorning snack to keep your energy levels up. (Got an egg allergy? No problem. Simply skip the protein powder. They are equally delicious without it.)

INGREDIENTS

1¼ cups walnuts

1 cup dried apricots

⅓ cup almonds, sliced

⅓ cup egg white protein powder

¼ cup water

SUPPLIES

measuring cups

food processor

baking dish

Place the walnuts in a food processor and pulse for about 20 seconds, or until granular.

Add the apricots, almonds, protein powder, and water and pulse for about 45 seconds, or until thoroughly combined.

Scoop out the mixture and press into a square or rectangular baking dish. An 8-inch square dish makes 10 to 12, ½-inch-thick bars.

Cut into your desired serving size and place the dish in the refrigerator to set for about an hour.

Once set, serve immediately or keep refrigerated and snack on these bars throughout the week.

Maca Superfood Bars

Superfoods have been the topic of the century, only very few people are actually listening. To optimize your health, it pays to consume superfoods, daily and these bars will get you well on your way to super-health. This bar incorporates chia seeds and Maca powder, South American secrets for a natural energy boost. (If you have an egg allergy, simply skip the protein powder.)

INGREDIENTS

1¼ cups walnuts

1 cup dried apples

½ cup raisins

¼ cup chia seeds

½ teaspoon Maca powder

⅓ cup egg white protein powder

¼ cup water

SUPPLIES

measuring cups

food processor

baking dish

Place the walnuts in a food processor and pulse for about 20 seconds, or until granular.

Add the apples, raisins, chia seeds, Maca powder, protein powder, and water, and pulse for about 45 seconds, or until thoroughly combined.

Scoop out the mixture and press into a square or rectangular baking dish. An 8x8-inch dish makes 10 to 12, half-inch-thick bars.

Cut into your desired serving size and place the dish in the refrigerator to set for about an hour.

Once set, serve immediately or keep refrigerated and snack on these bars throughout the week.

Chia Chocolate Superfood Bars

Chia seeds have recently become popularized and now appear on the shelves of many health stores. They have been consumed in South America for centuries as a great source of energy and fatty acids. Combined with cacao powder, the bars are both delicious and nutrient-dense. (As always, you can skip the protein if you have an egg allergy.)

INGREDIENTS

1¼ cups walnuts

1 cup dried apples

¼ cup chia seeds

¼ cup cacao powder

⅓ cup egg white protein powder

¼ cup water

SUPPLIES

measuring cups

food processor

baking dish

Place the walnuts in a food processor and pulse for about 20 seconds, or until granular.

Add the apples, chia seeds, cacao powder, protein powder, and water, and pulse for about 45 seconds, or until thoroughly combined.

Scoop out the mixture and press into a square or rectangular baking dish. An 8x8-inch dish makes 10 to 12, half-inch-thick bars.

Cut into your desired serving size and place the dish in the refrigerator to set for about an hour.

Once set, serve immediately or keep refrigerated and snack on these bars throughout the week.

Chocolate Orange Superfood Bar

Rich in antioxidants and delicately flavored to taste like a chocolate-orange treat, these bars make a great snack anytime you need a boost or have a chocolate craving. (Substitute the protein powder with Maca powder if you have an egg allergy.)

INGREDIENTS

1¼ cups walnuts

1 cup dried apples

¼ cup cacao powder

¼ cup grated orange zest

⅓ cup egg white protein powder

¼ cup water

SUPPLIES

measuring cups

food processor

baking dish

Place the walnuts in a food processor and pulse for about 20 seconds, or until granular.

Add the apples, cacao powder, orange zest, protein powder, and water, and pulse for about 45 seconds, or until thoroughly combined.

Scoop out the mixture and press into a square or rectangular baking dish. An 8x8-inch dish makes 10 to 12, half-inch-thick bars.

Cut into your desired serving size and place the dish in the refrigerator to set for about an hour.

Once set, serve immediately or keep refrigerated and snack on these bars throughout the week.

Acai Pomegranate Superfood Bar

High in vitamin A, vitamin C, and fatty acid, acai berries have become all the craze and for good reason. (Substitute the protein powder with Maca powder if you have an egg allergy.)

INGREDIENTS

1¼ cups walnuts

1 cup dried apples

¼ cup dried acai berries

¼ cup dried pomegranate seeds

½ teaspoon cacao powder

⅓ cup egg white protein powder

¼ cup water

SUPPLIES

measuring cups

food processor

baking dish

Place the walnuts in a food processor and pulse for about 20 seconds, or until granular.

Add the apples, berries, pomegranate seeds, cacao powder, protein powder, and water and pulse for about 45 seconds, or until thoroughly combined.

Scoop out the mixture and press into a square or rectangular baking dish. An 8x8-inch dish makes 10 to 12, half-inch-thick bars.

Cut into your desired serving size and place the dish in the refrigerator to set for about an hour.

Once set, serve immediately or keep refrigerated and snack on these bars throughout the week.

Maca Goji Superfood Bar

Known as one of the most nutrient-rich foods on earth, goji berries are considered a complete protein and are home to more than 20 trace minerals. These bars are a great option to get you through a strenuous workout. (Simply leave out the protein powder if you have an egg allergy.)

INGREDIENTS

1¼ cups walnuts

1 cup dried apples

½ cup dried goji berries

½ teaspoon Maca powder

⅓ cup egg white protein powder

¼ cup water

SUPPLIES

measuring cups and spoon

food processor

baking dish

Place the walnuts in a food processor and pulse for about 20 seconds, or until granular.

Add the apples, goji berries, Maca powder, protein powder, and water, and pulse for about 45 seconds, or until thoroughly combined.

Scoop out the mixture and press into a square or rectangular baking dish. An 8x8-inch dish makes 10 to 12, half-inch-thick bars.

Cut into your desired serving size and place the dish in the refrigerator to set for about an hour.

Once set, serve immediately or keep refrigerated and snack on these bars throughout the week.

TIP: If ever your bars turn out too sticky for your liking, simply sprinkle unsweetened coconut flakes over the cut squares before refrigerating.

Banana Smoothie

Bananas offer an excellent dose of vitamin B6 and natural potassium. Added to smoothies, they provide nutrients and form the perfect base for adding superfoods and natural flavors. (Substitute the protein powder with Maca powder if you have an egg allergy.)

INGREDIENTS

ice

½ cup coconut milk

1 banana

¼ cup egg white protein powder

½ teaspoon cinnamon powder

SUPPLIES

measuring cups and spoon

blender

serving glass or to-go cup

Add the ice to the blender.

Pour the coconut milk over the ice.

Add the peeled banana and protein powder, and blend until the ice is fully crushed.

Pour into a tall glass, sprinkle cinnamon on top, and enjoy.

Chocolate Smoothie

Antioxidant-packed and delicious, this smoothie will satisfy any sweet tooth craving. (Substitute the protein powder with Maca powder if you have an egg allergy.)

INGREDIENTS

ice

½ cup coconut milk

1 banana

¼ cup egg white protein powder

⅛ cup cacao powder

½ teaspoon cinnamon powder

SUPPLIES

measuring cups and spoons

blender

serving glass or to-go cup

Add the ice to the blender.

Pour the coconut milk over the ice.

Add the peeled banana, protein powder, and cacao powder, and blend until the ice is fully crushed.

Pour into a tall glass, sprinkle the cinnamon on top, and enjoy.

Chocolate Orange Smoothie

Add orange to the chocolate-lover's dream. If you love orange chocolate, this smoothie is for you. (Substitute the protein powder with Maca powder if you have an egg allergy.)

INGREDIENTS

ice

½ cup coconut milk

1 banana

¼ cup egg white protein powder

2 tablespoons cacao powder

½ orange, squeezed

½ teaspoon cinnamon powder

SUPPLIES

measuring cups and spoons

blender

serving glass or to-go cup

Add the ice to the blender.

Pour the coconut milk over the ice.

Add the peeled banana, protein powder, cacao powder, and freshly squeezed orange juice, and blend until the ice is fully crushed.

Pour into a tall glass, sprinkle cinnamon on top, and enjoy.

Lime Smoothie

Refreshing and light, this smoothie is a great morning pick-me-up or tropical drink for a poolside getaway. (Substitute the protein powder with Maca powder if you have an egg allergy.)

INGREDIENTS

ice

½ cup coconut milk

1 banana

¼ cup egg white protein powder

1 lime, squeezed

½ teaspoon cinnamon powder

SUPPLIES

measuring cups and spoon

blender

serving glass or to-go cup

Add the ice to the blender.

Pour the coconut milk over the ice.

Add the peeled banana, protein powder, and freshly squeezed lime juice, and blend until the ice is fully crushed.

Pour into a tall glass, sprinkle cinnamon on top, and enjoy.

Green Mamba Smoothie

Spirulina, from natural algae, is a superfood that is extremely rich in protein and, combined with kale, is dense in vitamins A, C, and K, providing a great start to any day. (Substitute the protein powder with Maca powder if you have an egg allergy.)

INGREDIENTS

ice

½ cup coconut milk

1 banana

¼ cup egg white protein powder

½ cup chopped kale

1 tablespoon spirulina powder

½ teaspoon cinnamon powder

SUPPLIES

measuring cups and spoons

blender

serving glass or to-go cup

Add the ice to the blender.

Pour the coconut milk over the ice.

Add the peeled banana, protein powder, kale, and spirulina powder, and blend until the ice is fully crushed.

Pour into a tall glass, sprinkle cinnamon on top, and enjoy.

Bonus

Enjoy your smoothies with pearls? Try adding chia seeds instead of the traditional tapioca pearl "bubbles" for a superfood enhancement that's rich in omegas.

Easy Morning Muffins

This is the simplest muffin recipe (probably ever!), allowing you to whip up delicious muffins in no time at all. They are protein-rich, so they make a great addition to breakfast, or an excellent snack any time of the day.

INGREDIENTS

½ cup dried apricots

¼ cup coconut flour

½ cup coconut oil, melted

1 shake salt

¼ teaspoon baking soda

4 eggs

½ teaspoon honey

⅛ teaspoon vanilla extract

SUPPLIES

measuring cups and spoons

food processor

muffin liners (optional)

muffin tin

Preheat the oven to 325°F.

Place muffin liners in the muffin tin or lightly grease a muffin tin.

Add the apricots to the food processor and pulse until finely chopped.

Add the rest of the ingredients to the food processor and pulse for about 2 minutes, or until well combined.

Scoop 2 tablespoons of the mixture into each muffin liner, or into a greased muffin tin and bake for about 14 minutes, or until a skewer poked through the center comes out clean.

Remove from the oven and allow to cool for a few minutes before serving, or refrigerate and enjoy within 5 days.

Raspberry Zucchini Muffins

There is nothing quite like a muffin in the morning, and the best thing about these muffins is they'll fill you up and won't make you crash! Plus, raspberries are high in antioxidants and zucchini gives you a morning dose of vegetables.

INGREDIENTS

¼ cup coconut oil + more for greasing

1 cup almond flour

1 teaspoon baking soda

¼ teaspoon salt (optional)

grated zest of ¼ orange

1 cup almond butter

2 eggs

⅓ cup honey

⅓ cup almond slices

½ cup grated zucchini

½ pint raspberries

SUPPLIES

measuring cups and spoons

muffin liners (optional)

muffin tin

2 medium mixing bowls

spatula

Preheat the oven to 350°F.

Place muffin liners in the muffin tin or lightly grease a muffin tin with coconut oil.

Mix the dry ingredients together in a mixing bowl.

Mix the wet ingredients together in another bowl.

Combine the dry and wet ingredients in one bowl.

Fold in the raspberries (raspberries should be left whole).

Scoop the batter into the muffin liners or muffin tin and bake for 15 to 20 minutes or until a skewer poked through the center comes out clean.

Remove from the oven and allow to cool for a few minutes before serving.

Note: If you're using an egg substitute, the muffins may not rise as much as they would with eggs, but they're just as tasty!

Pumpkin Muffins

Packed with fall flavors, pumpkin muffins are tasty and a great substitute for pumpkin bread during your Thanksgiving meal.

INGREDIENTS

¼ cup coconut oil + more for greasing

1 teaspoon cinnamon powder

1 teaspoon allspice powder

1 cup almond flour

1 teaspoon baking soda

¼ teaspoon salt (optional)

½ teaspoon almond extract

1 cup almond butter

2 eggs

⅓ cup honey

⅓ cup almond slices

½ cup baked pumpkin (or canned pumpkin)

½ cup grated zucchini

SUPPLIES

measuring cups and spoons

muffin liners (optional)

muffin tin

2 medium mixing bowls

Preheat the oven to 350°F.

Place muffin liners in the muffin tin or lightly grease a muffin tin with coconut oil.

Mix the dry ingredients together in a mixing bowl.

Mix the wet ingredients together in another bowl.

Combine the dry and wet ingredients in one bowl.

Scoop the batter into the muffin liners or muffin tin and bake for 15 to 20 minutes or until a skewer poked through the center comes out clean.

Remove from the oven and allow to cool for a few minutes before serving.

Note: If you're using an egg substitute, the muffins may not rise as much as they would with eggs, but they're just as tasty!

Orange Muffins

Get your vitamin C in this great muffin form!

INGREDIENTS

¼ cup coconut oil + more for greasing

1 cup almond flour

1 teaspoon baking soda

¼ teaspoon salt (optional)

¾ to 1 teaspoon grated orange zest

1 cup almond butter

2 eggs

⅓ cup honey

⅓ cup almond slices

½ cup grated zucchini

SUPPLIES

measuring cups and spoons

muffin liners (optional)

muffin tin

2 medium mixing bowls

Preheat the oven to 350°F.

Place muffin liners in the muffin tin or lightly grease a muffin tin with coconut oil.

Mix the dry ingredients together in a mixing bowl.

Mix the wet ingredients together in another bowl.

Combine the dry and wet ingredients in one bowl.

Scoop the batter into the muffin liners or muffin tin and bake for 15 to 20 minutes or until a skewer poked through the center comes out clean.

Remove from the oven and allow to cool for a few minutes before serving.

Note: If you're using an egg substitute, the muffins may not rise as much as they would with eggs, but they're just as tasty!

Banana Muffins

Bananas make anything rich and moist, so these muffins will melt in your mouth. Plus, you're getting your potassium.

INGREDIENTS
¼ cup coconut oil + more for greasing

1 cup almond flour

1 teaspoon baking soda

¼ teaspoon salt (optional)

½ teaspoon almond extract

1 cup almond butter

2 eggs

⅓ cup honey

⅓ cup walnuts

1 banana, mashed

½ cup grated zucchini

SUPPLIES
measuring cups and spoons

muffin liners (optional)

muffin tin

2 medium mixing bowls

Preheat the oven to 350°F.

Place muffin liners in the muffin tin or lightly grease a muffin tin with coconut oil.

Mix the dry ingredients together in a mixing bowl.

Mix the wet ingredients together in another bowl.

Combine the dry and wet ingredients in one bowl.

Scoop the batter into the muffin liners or muffin tin and bake for 15 to 20 minutes or until a skewer poked through the center comes out clean.

Remove from the oven and allow to cool for a few minutes before serving.

Note: If you're using an egg substitute, the muffins may not rise as much as they would with eggs, but they're just as tasty!

Blackberry Muffins

High in dietary fiber, vitamin K, and vitamin C, blackberries are a delicious addition to any baking product.

INGREDIENTS

¼ cup coconut oil + more for greasing

1 cup almond flour

1 teaspoon baking soda

¼ teaspoon salt (optional)

½ teaspoon grated orange zest

1 cup almond butter

2 eggs

⅓ cup honey

⅓ cup almond slices

½ cup grated zucchini

½ pint blackberries

SUPPLIES

measuring cups

muffin liners (optional)

muffin tin

2 medium mixing bowls

spatula

Preheat the oven to 350°F.

Place muffin liners in the muffin tin or lightly grease a muffin tin with coconut oil.

Mix the dry ingredients together in a mixing bowl.

Mix the wet ingredients together in another bowl.

Combine the dry and wet ingredients in one bowl.

Fold in the blackberries (blackberries should be left whole).

Scoop the batter into the muffin liners or muffin tin and bake for 15 to 20 minutes or until a skewer poked through the center comes out clean.

Remove from the oven and allow to cool for a few minutes before serving.

Note: If you're using an egg substitute the muffins may not rise as much as they would with eggs, but they're just as tasty!

Hearty Traditional Breakfast

Who doesn't love a traditional breakfast?! The good news is that on the Paleo Diet you can enjoy one every day, without the guilt.

INGREDIENTS

½ tablespoon coconut oil

2 strips bacon

1 egg

¼ cup coconut milk

½ tomato, diced

¼ cup spinach, chopped

½ teaspoon dried basil

measuring cups and spoons

sharp knife

medium mixing bowl

large sauté pan

Heat the coconut oil in a large sauté pan over medium heat until it liquefies.

Place the bacon strips to one side of the pan.

In a bowl, beat the egg, coconut milk, tomato, spinach, and basil until combined.

Pour the mixture into the pan alongside the bacon (the omelet absorbs the bacon flavor).

Flip and cook until done to your liking, then enjoy everything hot.

Bonus

Add one (or more!) of the below items as a side dish to go with your hearty traditional breakfast for even more nutrients and to further tantalize your taste buds.

Add Grilled Banana

INGREDIENTS

1 teaspoon coconut oil

1 banana

cinnamon powder

SUPPLIES

measuring spoon

sharp knife

sauté pan

Melt the coconut oil in a sauté pan over medium heat.

Slice the banana down the middle and place both halves in the pan to grill, flipping over after about a minute.

Grill until soft, then remove from the pan and add cinnamon to taste.

Add Garlic Mushrooms

INGREDIENTS

1 teaspoon coconut oil

5 button mushrooms, thinly sliced

1 clove garlic, finely chopped

dried oregano

SUPPLIES

measuring spoon

sharp knife

sauté pan

Melt the coconut oil in a sauté pan over medium heat.

Add the mushrooms and garlic to the pan to sauté, stirring periodically.

Cook until slightly browned, then remove from the pan and add oregano to taste.

Add Breakfast Sausage

INGREDIENTS

1 teaspoon coconut oil

¼ pound breakfast sausage

1 tablespoon black pepper

1 tablespoon honey

SUPPLIES

measuring spoons

medium mixing bowl

sauté pan

Melt the coconut oil in a sauté pan over medium heat.

In a mixing bowl, combine the sausage, pepper, and honey with your hands and form into your desired patty size.

Place the patty in the pan to cook for about 4 minutes (depending on thickness), flipping every minute.

Cook until well done, then remove from the pan and serve hot.

Add Grilled Tomato

INGREDIENTS

1 tablespoon coconut oil

1 tomato, sliced in half

dried oregano

SUPPLIES

measuring spoon

sharp knife

sauté pan

Melt the coconut oil in a sauté pan over medium heat.

Add the tomato halves to the pan to cook for about 4 minutes, flipping after 2 minutes.

Cook until soft, then remove from the pan and add oregano to taste.

Super Snacks

It's 10 a.m. and you're hungry. That's okay; just don't reach for the carbs! There are plenty of super-easy and super-delicious Paleo snacks you can premake or whip together in no time at all to put your snack attacks at bay.

Guacamole

An extremely easy option for a snack is guacamole, paired with carrots and celery sticks for dipping.

INGREDIENTS

1 avocado

1 lime

¼ teaspoon salt (optional)

¼ teaspoon black pepper

1 seeded and diced jalapeño

1 tablespoon garlic powder

SUPPLIES

measuring cups and spoons

sharp knife

medium mixing bowl

Extract the flesh from the avocado and place in the mixing bowl.

Cut lime and squeeze the juice on top of the avocado.

Add the salt, pepper, jalapeño, and garlic to the avocado mix and mash together thoroughly before serving.

Flax Raisin Loaf

A wholesome snack that pairs extremely well with the Paleo hummus recipes we introduced you to during the Paleo Cleanse.

INGREDIENTS

3 tablespoons coconut oil, divided

2¼ cups golden flax meal

3 tablespoons coconut flour

½ teaspoon baking soda

1 teaspoon cinnamon, powder

¼ teaspoon salt

½ cup coconut milk

4 eggs

¼ cup water

¼ cup honey

1 tablespoon apple cider vinegar

¾ cup raisins

SUPPLIES

measuring cups and spoons

8x5 inch bread pan

food processor

spatula

Preheat the oven to 350°F.

Grease a bread pan with 1 tablespoon of coconut oil.

Place the flax meal, coconut flour, baking soda, cinnamon, and salt in a food processor, and pulse for about 20 seconds, or until mixed.

Add the coconut milk, eggs, water, honey, apple cider vinegar, and the other 2 tablespoons of coconut oil to the food processor and pulse until well blended.

Fold in the raisins.

Scoop the mixture into the greased bread pan and place in the oven to bake for about 35 minutes, or until a skewer poked through the center comes out clean.

Remove from the oven and let cool before slicing.

Flax Apricot Loaf

Adding apricots to the flaxseed loaf boosts an already fiber-filled recipe!

INGREDIENTS

3 tablespoons coconut oil, divided

2¼ cups golden flax meal

3 tablespoons coconut flour

½ teaspoon baking soda

¼ teaspoon salt

½ cup coconut milk

4 eggs

¼ cup water

¼ cup honey

1 tablespoon apple cider vinegar

½ cup dried apricots

SUPPLIES

measuring cups

8x5 inch bread pan

food processor

spatula

Preheat the oven to 350°F.

Grease a bread pan with 1 tablespoon of coconut oil.

Place the flax meal, coconut flour, baking soda, and salt in a food processor, and pulse for about 20 seconds, or until mixed.

Add the coconut milk, eggs, water, honey, apple cider vinegar, dried apricots, and the other 2 tablespoons of coconut oil to the food processor and pulse until well blended.

Scoop the mixture into the greased bread pan and place in the oven to bake for about 35 minutes, or until a skewer poked through the center comes out clean.

Remove from the oven and let cool before slicing.

Flax Cranberry Orange Loaf

INGREDIENTS

3 tablespoons coconut oil, divided

2¼ cups golden flax meal

3 tablespoons coconut flour

½ teaspoon baking soda

¼ teaspoon salt

½ cup coconut milk

4 eggs

¼ cup water

¼ cup honey

1 tablespoon apple cider vinegar

½ cup unsweetened dried cranberries

grated zest of 1 orange

SUPPLIES

measuring cups and spoons

8x5 inch bread pan

food processor

spatula

Preheat the oven to 350°F.

Grease a bread pan with 1 tablespoon of coconut oil.

Place the flax meal, coconut flour, baking soda, and salt in a food processor and pulse for about 20 seconds, or until mixed.

Add the coconut milk, eggs, water, honey, apple cider vinegar, dried cranberries, orange rind, and the other 2 tablespoons of coconut oil to the food processor and pulse until well blended.

Scoop the mixture into the greased bread pan and place in the oven to bake for about 35 minutes, or until a skewer poked through the center comes out clean.

Remove from the oven and let cool before slicing.

Flax Banana Loaf

The addition of banana makes the traditional flaxseed loaf moist and fluffy.

INGREDIENTS

3 tablespoons coconut oil, divided

2¼ cups golden flax meal

3 tablespoons coconut flour

½ teaspoon baking soda

¼ teaspoon salt

1 teaspoon nutmeg powder

½ cup coconut milk

4 eggs

¼ cup water

¼ cup honey

1 tablespoon apple cider vinegar

1 ripe banana

SUPPLIES

measuring cups and spoons

8x5 inch bread pan

food processor

spatula

Preheat the oven to 350°F.

Grease a bread pan with 1 tablespoon of coconut oil.

Place the flax meal, coconut flour, baking soda, salt, and nutmeg in a food processor, and pulse for about 20 seconds, or until mixed.

Add the coconut milk, eggs, water, honey, apple cider vinegar, banana, and the other 2 tablespoons of coconut oil to the food processor and pulse until well blended.

Scoop the mixture into the greased bread pan and place in the oven to bake for about 35 minutes, or until a skewer poked through the center comes out clean.

Remove from the oven and let cool before slicing.

Bonus

Make any of the above flax bread recipes into muffins instead of loaves. Simply scoop the mixture into muffin liners or a greased muffin tin instead of the bread pan and bake for about 25 minutes.

Raisin Bread

The sweet scent of freshly baked bread and the satisfaction of
a hearty, homemade loaf add to the appeal of this recipe. It's
foolproof and will have you baking loaves week in and week out.

INGREDIENTS

2 tablespoons coconut oil, divided

2 cups arrowroot flour

½ cup flax meal

¼ cup coconut flour

½ teaspoon baking soda

¼ teaspoon salt

5 eggs

1 tablespoon apple cider vinegar

1 tablespoon honey

¾ cup raisins

SUPPLIES

measuring cups and spoons

8x5 inch bread pan

food processor

spatula

Preheat the oven to 350°F.

Grease a bread pan with 1 tablespoon of coconut oil.

In a food processor, add the arrowroot, flax meal, coconut flour, baking
soda, and salt, and pulse for about 1 minute.

Add the eggs, other tablespoon of coconut oil, apple cider vinegar, and
honey, and blend for about another minute.

Fold in the raisins.

Scoop the mixture into the greased bread pan and bake for 35 to 40
minutes, or until a skewer poked through the center of the loaf comes
out clean.

Remove from the oven and let cool before slicing.

Apricot Apple Raisin Bread

Fiber-packed and naturally sweet to help you fight any sugar cravings!

INGREDIENTS

2 tablespoons coconut oil, divided

2 cups arrowroot flour

½ cup flax meal

¼ cup coconut flour

½ teaspoon baking soda

¼ teaspoon salt

5 eggs

1 tablespoon apple cider vinegar

⅓ cup dried apricots

½ cup dried apples

1 tablespoon honey

½ cup raisins

SUPPLIES

measuring cups and spoons

8x5 inch bread pan

food processor

spatula

Preheat the oven to 350°F.

Grease a bread pan with 1 tablespoon of coconut oil.

In a food processor, add the arrowroot, flax meal, coconut flour, baking soda, and salt, and pulse for about 1 minute.

Add the eggs, other tablespoon of coconut oil, apple cider vinegar, apricots, apples, and honey and blend for about another minute.

Fold in the raisins.

Scoop the mixture into the greased bread pan and bake for 35 to 40 minutes, or until a skewer poked through the center of the loaf comes out clean.

Remove from the oven and let cool before slicing.

Cranberry Orange Bread

Zest and spice and everything nice!

INGREDIENTS
2 tablespoons coconut oil, divided

2 cups arrowroot flour

½ cup flax meal

¼ cup coconut flour

½ teaspoon baking soda

¼ teaspoon salt

5 eggs

1 tablespoon apple cider vinegar

grated zest of 1 orange

1 tablespoon honey

½ cup unsweetened dried cranberries

SUPPLIES
measuring cups and spoons

8x5 inch bread pan

food processor

spatula

Preheat the oven to 350°F.

Grease a bread pan with 1 tablespoon of coconut oil.

In a food processor, add the arrowroot flour, flax meal, coconut flour, baking soda, and salt, and pulse for about 1 minute.

Add the eggs, second tablespoon of coconut oil, apple cider vinegar, orange zest, and honey, and blend for about another minute.

Fold in the cranberries.

Scoop the mixture into the greased bread pan and bake for 35 to 40 minutes, or until a skewer poked through the center of the loaf comes out clean.

Remove from the oven and let cool before slicing.

Anise Seed Raisin Bread

Get the wheat flavor without the side effects!

INGREDIENTS

2 tablespoons coconut oil, divided

2 cups arrowroot flour

½ cup flax meal

¼ cup coconut flour

½ teaspoon baking soda

¼ teaspoon salt

5 eggs

1 tablespoon apple cider vinegar

1 tablespoon honey

¾ cup raisins

¼ cup anise seeds

SUPPLIES

measuring cups and spoons

8x5 inch bread pan

food processor

spatula

Preheat the oven to 350°F.

Grease a bread pan with 1 tablespoon of coconut oil.

In a food processor, add the arrowroot flour, flax meal, coconut flour, baking soda, and salt, and pulse for about 1 minute.

Add the eggs, other tablespoon of coconut oil, apple cider vinegar, and honey, and blend for about another minute.

Fold in the raisins and anise seeds.

Scoop the mixture into the greased bread pan and bake for 35 to 40 minutes, or until a skewer poked through the center of the loaf comes out clean.

Remove from the oven and let cool before slicing.

Walnut Raisin Bread

This recipe is rich in natural fats to nourish your body.

INGREDIENTS

2 tablespoons coconut oil, divided

2 cups arrowroot flour

½ cup flax meal

¼ cup coconut flour

½ teaspoon baking soda

¼ teaspoon salt

5 eggs

1 tablespoon apple cider vinegar

1 tablespoon honey

⅓ cup walnuts, chopped

¾ cup raisins

SUPPLIES

measuring cups and spoons

8x5 inch bread pan

food processor

spatula

Preheat the oven to 350°F.

Grease a bread pan with 1 tablespoon of coconut oil.

In a food processor, add the arrowroot flour, flax meal, coconut flour, baking soda, and salt, and pulse for about 1 minute.

Add the eggs, second tablespoon of coconut oil, apple cider vinegar, and honey, and blend for about another minute.

Fold in the walnuts and raisins.

Scoop the mixture into the greased bread pan and bake for 35 to 40 minutes, or until a skewer poked through the center of the loaf comes out clean.

Remove from the oven and let cool before slicing.

Sweet Chili Jerky

If you enjoyed the jerky recipes from the Paleo Cleanse *Meal Plans*, you might like to try this twist on the classic.

INGREDIENTS

1 (4–5 pound) frozen beef roast

1 cup honey

⅓ cup balsamic vinegar

2 teaspoons red pepper flakes

⅓ cup pineapple juice

2 teaspoons black pepper

1 tablespoon onion powder

1 teaspoon salt

SUPPLIES

measuring cups and spoons

sharp knife

deep bowl

mixing bowl

aluminum foil

baking sheet

Place the frozen roast out to defrost until the outside rim of the roast is soft but the center is still slightly frozen.

Slice the roast into strips that are about ⅛-inch thick and place the strips in a bowl.

Combine the honey, vinegar, red pepper flakes, pineapple juice, black pepper, and onion powder in a bowl and mix to form the marinade.

Pour the marinade over the beef strips.

Sprinkle with salt and stir until the marinade coats all the beef.

Allow the mixture to sit and marinate for at least 2 hours (overnight in the refrigerator is better if time allows).

Preheat the oven to 190°F.

Place the beef strips onto a foil-lined baking sheet.

Place in the oven to bake and flip about every 30 minutes.

To test if the jerky is done, fold a piece in half and look for white threads. If you see white threads, the jerky is cooked.

Once done, remove the jerky from the oven and allow to cool before serving, or refrigerate and enjoy within 5 days.

TIP: Make sure you cut the jerky thin enough—otherwise you'll get little, not-so-tasty steaks. Also, having the meat slightly frozen will make it easier to cut. Use a serrated knife and keep hot water running to run your hands under—they will get cold!

Garlic Jerky

Another tweak to our classic homemade jerky
recipe, this one embraces the love of garlic.

INGREDIENTS

1 (4–5 pound) frozen beef roast

1 clove garlic, crushed

1 (10-ounce) bottle balsamic vinegar

2 tablespoons onion powder

1 teaspoon salt

SUPPLIES

measuring spoons

sharp knife

marinade bowl

aluminum foil

baking sheet

Place the frozen roast out to defrost until the outside rim of the roast is soft but the center is still slightly frozen.

Slice the roast into strips that are about ⅛-inch thick and place the strips in a bowl.

Combine the garlic, vinegar, and onion powder in a bowl and mix to form the marinade.

Pour the marinade over the beef strips.

Sprinkle with salt and stir until the marinade coats all the beef.

Allow the mixture to sit and marinate for at least 2 hours (overnight in the refrigerator is better if time allows).

Preheat the oven to 190°F.

Place the beef strips onto a foil-lined baking sheet.

Place in the oven to bake and flip about every 30 minutes.

To test if the jerky is done, fold a piece in half and look for white threads. If you see white threads, the jerky is cooked.

One done, remove the jerky from the oven and allow to cool before serving, or refrigerate and enjoy within 5 days.

Bonus

Switch up the flavor a little by using bison or deer meat instead of beef. When using deer, allow the meat to marinate longer to reduce the game flavor.

Convenient Lunches

Who has time to prepare elaborate lunches during the week? We know that quick and easy is the key to ensuring healthy midday dining. Enjoy these convenient recipes so you stay on track despite your busy schedule.

Tuna Salad

This is a fast and easy recipe, and is the perfect healthy option for when you don't have time to slave over the stovetop.

INGREDIENTS

3 leaves romaine

1 (2.5-ounce) pack tuna (wheat- and soy-free)

½ cucumber, diced

¼ red onion, diced

¼ cup cherry tomatoes, diced

¼ cup olive tapenade (vegetable oil-, wheat- and soy-free)

2 tablespoons red wine vinegar

SUPPLIES

measuring cups and spoon

sharp knife

small mixing bowl

Rinse the lettuce and rip into small sections before placing in a bowl.

Drain the tuna and place it in the bowl on top of the lettuce.

Add the cucumber, red onion, cherry tomatoes, olive tapenade, and vinegar to the bowl and then mix all the ingredients.

Refrigerate and enjoy within a day.

Steak Salad

The perfect combination of protein and fresh greens, this salad makes for a great energy-sustaining lunch.

INGREDIENTS

3 leaves romaine

4 to 5 slices cooked steak

2 tablespoons olive oil

1 tablespoon red wine

½ cucumber, diced

¼ red onion, diced

¼ cup cherry tomatoes, diced

¼ cup olive tapenade (vegetable oil-, wheat- and soy-free)

SUPPLIES

measuring cups and spoon

sharp knife

small mixing bowl

shaker

Rinse the lettuce and rip into small sections before placing in a bowl.

Heat the steak strips and place them in the bowl on top of the lettuce.

Place the olive oil and red wine in the shaker and shake for about 20 seconds.

Add the cucumber, red onion, cherry tomatoes, and olive tapenade to the bowl.

Drizzle with olive oil and red wine blend.

Toss and serve.

Chicken Salad

Light yet protein-rich, this recipe is great as a main course or as a filling between two slices of Paleo Bread.

INGREDIENTS

3 leaves romaine

¼ pound cooked chicken breast, sliced into strips

½ cucumber, diced

¼ red onion, diced

¼ cup cherry tomatoes, diced

¼ cup olive tapenade (vegetable oil-, wheat- and soy-free)

2 tablespoons balsamic vinegar

SUPPLIES

measuring cups and spoon

sharp knife

small mixing bowl

Rinse the lettuce and rip into small sections before placing in a bowl.

Place the chicken strips in the bowl on top of the lettuce.

Add the cucumber, red onion, cherry tomatoes, olive tapenade, and vinegar to the bowl and then mix all the ingredients.

Refrigerate and enjoy within a day.

Summer Salad

Full of antioxidants and vitamins, this summer salad is
as refreshing and nutrient-dense as it is tasty.

INGREDIENTS

1 cup spinach leaves

½ cucumber, diced

¼ red onion, diced

½ cup walnuts, chopped

½ cup strawberries, sliced

2 tablespoons red wine vinegar

SUPPLIES

measuring cups and spoon

sharp knife

small mixing bowl

Place the spinach, cucumber, onion, walnuts, and strawberries in a bowl.

Add the vinegar to the bowl and then mix all the ingredients.

Serve immediately and enjoy.

Meatless Spaghetti Sauce

Free of vegetable oils common in store-bought spaghetti
sauce, this recipe is easy and full of flavor. Pair with
almond flour pasta, or serve over vegetables.

INGREDIENTS

1 tablespoon coconut oil

1 yellow onion, diced

1 large carrot, chopped

1 (28- to 32-ounce) can crushed tomatoes

3 cloves garlic, crushed

1 tablespoon black pepper

2 tablespoons Italian seasoning

1 teaspoon salt (optional)

SUPPLIES

measuring spoons

sharp knife

medium pot

Melt the coconut oil in a pot over medium-high heat.

Add the onion and carrot to the pot and cook until the onion starts to brown.

Add the tomatoes, garlic, pepper, Italian seasoning, and salt, then reduce the heat to medium and cover the pan.

Cook for at least 20 minutes before serving hot.

Spaghetti Sauce with Meat

Enjoy a taste of Italy, without the breadcrumbs common in store-bought meat sauce. Serve with almond flour pasta, or over vegetables.

INGREDIENTS

1 tablespoon coconut oil

1 yellow onion, diced

1 large carrot, chopped

1 (28- to 32-ounce) can crushed tomatoes

3 cloves garlic, crushed

1 tablespoon black pepper

2 tablespoons Italian seasoning

1 teaspoon salt (optional)

1 pound ground beef

SUPPLIES

measuring spoons

sharp knife

medium pot

Melt the coconut oil in a pot over medium-high heat.

Add the onion and carrot to the pot and cook until the onion starts to brown.

Add the tomatoes, garlic, pepper, Italian seasoning, salt, and beef, and let the mixture return to boil.

Once boiling, reduce the heat to medium and cover the pan.

Cook for about 45 minutes, stirring occasionally until the meat is cooked.

Serve hot.

Beef and Butternut Trifle

A simple dish made gourmet, this beef and butternut squash combination is hearty and filling, and is a great option for a dinner party.

INGREDIENTS
1 (2-pound) butternut squash, peeled and chopped into cubes

2 cloves garlic, chopped finely

½ cup diced fresh tomato

¼ cup sundried tomato, cut into thin slivers

1 tablespoon coconut oil

1 pound ground beef

dried oregano

SUPPLIES
measuring cups and spoon

sharp knife

large pot

large sauté pan

deep dish

In a large pot, bring water to a boil.

Add the butternut to the pot and cook for about 15 minutes, or until tender.

In a large pan, cook the garlic and the fresh and sundried tomatoes in the coconut oil over medium heat for about a minute, stirring occasionally.

Add the ground beef to the pan and cook until brown, stirring often.

Remove the butternut from the pot when cooked and mash.

In a deep dish, place a layer of mashed butternut followed by a layer of beef, then oregano spice. Repeat the layering; then serve hot.

Lime Chicken Wrap

Zest up any meal with this lean protein option, using your choice of lettuce wraps or coconut wraps.

INGREDIENTS

1 tablespoon coconut oil

¼ pound sliced chicken breast

1 teaspoon Cajun spice

½ lime, squeezed

lettuce leaves or coconut wraps

1 avocado

SUPPLIES

measuring spoons

sharp knife

medium sauté pan

Melt the coconut oil in a medium sauté pan over medium heat.

Season the chicken with Cajun spice, and cook the chicken in the pan with the lime juice over medium-high heat for about 10 minutes.

Scoop into the lettuce leaves or coconut wraps and top with avocado.

Drizzle with more lime juice before serving.

Ocean Wrap

Have fun with the taste of the ocean in this delectable wrap.

INGREDIENTS

1 tablespoon coconut oil

¼ pound halibut

1 clove garlic, chopped finely

salt

black pepper

lettuce leaves or coconut wraps

1 avocado

½ lemon, squeezed

SUPPLIES

measuring spoon

sharp knife

medium sauté pan

Melt the coconut oil in a medium sauté pan over medium heat.

Season the halibut with garlic, salt, and pepper, and cook the fish in the pan over medium-high heat for about 10 minutes.

Scoop into the leaves crowns or coconut wraps and top with avocado.

Drizzle with lemon before serving.

Apricot and Olive Chicken

Sweet, savory, and oh-so easy, this simple dish
makes enough for the whole family.

INGREDIENTS

2 tablespoons coconut oil

1 to 2 pounds chicken thighs/wings

½ cup apricots, sliced

⅓ cup olives stuffed with jalapeños, sliced

2 tablespoons honey

½ cup white wine

1½ teaspoons dried oregano

3 tablespoons red wine vinegar

6 cloves garlic, crushed

¼ teaspoon salt (optional)

¼ teaspoon black pepper

1 tablespoon capers

¼ cup parsley, chopped

SUPPLIES

measuring cups and spoons

sharp knife

medium sauté pan

slow cooker

Melt the coconut oil over medium-high heat in a sauté pan.

Cook the chicken until browned.

Place the apricots and olives into a slow cooker with the honey, white wine, oregano, vinegar, garlic, salt, black pepper, and capers.

Add the chicken and mix, then let it cook on high for about 1 hour.

Add the chopped parsley, cook for about 5 more minutes and enjoy hot.

Calamari Steak

Escape to the tropics with a seafood dish that's
tender, tasty, and high in omega-3.

INGREDIENTS

¼ cup arrowroot flour

½ pound calamari steak

2 tablespoon coconut oil, divided

1 tablespoon Cajun spice

½ lemon, squeezed

SUPPLIES

measuring cup and spoons

shallow medium bowl

medium sauté pan

Pour the flour into a shallow bowl.

Coat the calamari steak with 1 tablespoon of coconut oil then place in the flour, flipping to ensure both sides are coated.

In a sauté pan, heat the second tablespoon of coconut oil over medium heat and add the calamari. Cook until well-done.

Sprinkle with Cajun spice, top with lemon, and serve hot.

Spicy Chicken Wings

Turn up the heat with these chicken wings. They're perfect for any sports occasion or get-together.

INGREDIENTS

1 tablespoon ghee butter

8 chicken wings

3 cloves garlic, chopped finely

1 tablespoon finely chopped jalapeño

2 tablespoons paprika

SUPPLIES

measuring spoons

sharp knife

large sauté pan

In a large pan, heat the ghee butter over medium heat.

Add the chicken wings and cook for about 5 minutes, turning often.

Add the garlic and jalapeño and sprinkle with paprika.

Continue to cook on medium heat until well-done.

Place the chicken wings in a bowl and pour any remaining sauce from the pan over the top.

Serve hot.

Salad Dressings

Paleo Caesar Dressing

You don't have to give up Caesar dressing on the Paleo Diet. Enjoy this simple recipe free of soy and dairy that's so commonly found in store-bought salad dressings.

INGREDIENTS

¼ cup olive oil

1 tablespoon crushed garlic

1 tablespoon black pepper

1 lemon, squeezed

SUPPLIES

small mixing bowl

spoon

Pour the olive oil into the mixing bowl.

Add the garlic and black pepper and stir well.

Pour the lemon juice into the mix and stir briskly with a spoon before dressing a salad.

Citrus Dressing

A light and refreshing finish to a salad, this dressing recipe is as easy to make as it is delicious.

INGREDIENTS

¼ cup olive oil

¼ cup balsamic vinegar

1 orange, squeezed

SUPPLIES

small mixing bowl

spoon

Pour the olive oil and balsamic vinegar into the mixing bowl.

Add the orange juice and stir well with a spoon before dressing a salad.

Decadent Desserts

Life sometimes calls for sweeter moments; that's why we all need quick and easy Paleo dessert recipes on hand!

Coconut Sugar Cookies

Gluten-free cookies that will leave you wanting more!

INGREDIENTS

1 cup tapioca flour

¼ cup coconut flour

¼ teaspoon baking soda

½ teaspoon salt

½ cup grass-fed butter

½ cup coconut palm sugar

3 tablespoons water

1½ tablespoons honey

1 teaspoon vanilla extract

arrowroot flour, for rolling

¼ cup unsweetened coconut flakes

SUPPLIES

measuring cups and spoons

aluminum foil or parchment paper

baking sheet

food processor

rolling pin

cookie cutter

Preheat the oven to 325°F.

Place foil or parchment paper sheets over a baking sheet. This will prevent your cookies from sticking.

Combine the tapioca flour, coconut flour, baking soda, and salt in a small bowl.

In a food processor, pulse the butter and sugar for about 2 minutes, or until fluffy.

Add the dry ingredients, water, honey, and vanilla extract to the butter and sugar mixture and pulse until well combined.

Lightly dust arrowroot flour on a clean counter. Using a rolling pin, roll the cookie dough until 1/4-inch thick and then cut out your cookies using a cookie cutter.

Place the cookies on your lined baking sheet, sprinkle with coconut flakes, and bake for 12 to 14 minutes.

Remove from the oven and allow to cool for at least 10 minutes before serving.

Bonus

Like *The Paleo Pact* on Facebook to get your free copy of *Quick & Fantastic Paleo Cookies*, which includes ten other Paleo cookie recipes.

Dark Chocolate Brownies

Who doesn't love a chocolate brownie? Luckily there is a Paleo solution to this craving, and this recipe is decadent and filled with antioxidants and fiber.

INGREDIENTS

1 cup coconut flour

1/4 teaspoon baking soda

2 shakes salt

1.5 ounces dark chocolate, cubed

1/3 cup dark chocolate chips

7 dates, pitted

3 eggs

1/2 cup coconut oil, + more for greasing

1 teaspoon vanilla extract

SUPPLIES

measuring cups

food processor

baking dish

Preheat the oven to 350°F.

Pulse the flour, baking soda, and salt in a food processor.

Add the chocolate chips and the dates and pulse together until gritty.

Add the eggs, coconut oil, and vanilla extract, and pulse until well combined.

Scoop the mixture into a greased baking dish; a 6x6-inch pan makes thicker brownies, and an 8x8-inch pan makes for thinner bites. The mixture will be slightly spongy from the coconut flour, so press down firmly until evenly spread.

Place in the oven for about 20 minutes.

Remove from the oven and allow to cool.

Date Balls

As far as desserts go, this one's pretty good for you! Protein, dates, nuts, and the superfood qualities of cacao powder turn this delicious dessert into a guilt-free pleasure.

INGREDIENTS

2 tablespoons grass-fed butter

1 egg

1 tablespoon coconut palm sugar

1 tablespoon cacao powder

½ cup dates, pitted and chopped

½ cup walnuts, chopped

½ cup unsweetened coconut flakes

SUPPLIES

measuring cups

medium saucepan

mixing bowl

medium dish

In a medium saucepan, melt the grass-fed butter over low heat.

Add the egg, coconut palm sugar, and cacao powder to the pan and stir quickly until thoroughly blended.

Toss the dates and walnuts into a mixing bowl and pour in the heated mixture.

Stir until the mixture covers the dry ingredients.

Using your hands, form the mixture into bite-size dessert balls and hold each one together with a tiny sprinkle of coconut flakes.

Place in the refrigerator for about an hour to cool before serving.

Citrus Popsicle

Super easy to make, incredibly refreshing, and full of vitamin C, these frozen lollipops make a great summer dessert.

INGREDIENTS

2 tablespoons freshly squeezed orange juice

2 tablespoons freshly squeezed grapefruit juice

1 teaspoon honey

water (to fill ice pop mold)

SUPPLIES

measuring cups

ice pop mold

Pour all the ingredients into the ice pop mold and stir.

Seal the mold and place in the freezer until frozen.

CHAPTER 24

Final Thoughts

As we watch our generation and the generations succeeding us grow in size and disease rate, we have no choice but to start asking questions. Why were we lean, toned, and healthy millions of years ago when food was rudimentary, and now, despite our intelligence and advancements in technology, we are sicker than ever before?

Diet has an enormous impact on our bodies and our overall well-being. A diet based on industrial foods and refined sugar, with a high carbohydrate intake, fails to fuel the body with what it needs to be nourished and healthy.

Our health is the essence of our life. Good dietary choices are not optional—they are essential. Without our health we have nothing. With good health anything becomes possible!

As Abraham Lincoln so rightly said: "In the end, it's not the years in your life that count. It's the life in your years."

Congratulations once again on completing your Paleo Cleanse and for taking this journey with us. It has been an honor and we look forward to hearing your success stories.

To good health!

Camilla & Melissa

APPENDIX

Glossary

A glossary, because when you're trying something new it can be hard enough to keep track of the fundamentals.

Acai Berry—A berry that grows on a palm tree in the Brazilian rainforest. This type of berry is rich in nutrients and antioxidants and is considered a superfood.

Accountability Buddy—An individual to whom you are accountable. Someone who helps to keep you on track during your Cleanse.

Agave—A natural, low-glycemic sweetener that is derived from the agave plant.

All You Can Eat—The foods you can eat as much as you like of during the Paleo Cleanse.

Allergy or Allergies—A negative immune system response within the body, triggered by a foreign object.

Almond Flour—A Paleo-friendly flour that is made from ground almonds, also called almond meal.

Aloe Vera—Juice from the liliaceous plant, used to alkalize and detoxify.

Ancestors—The individuals from whom one has descended.

Ancestral Diet—A way of eating based upon the common diet of our ancestors and which we are evolutionary adapted to consume.

Antinutrients—Compounds that interfere with the body's natural absorption of nutrients.

Antioxidants—Organic substances that help to counteract and prevent the oxidation of tissues.

Arrowroot Flour—Flour that is derived from a tropical plant, often used for Paleo cooking.

Blood Sugar—The amount of sugar or glucose that is in your bloodstream at any given time. A large drop in blood sugar is commonly called a crash.

Cacao—A tropical tree that produces beans that can be processed into chocolate; considered to be a superfood.

Cage-Free—A term commonly used to describe certain eggs produced by birds who were not confined to a cage.

Carbohydrates—A class of chemical compounds that includes sugar and starches.

Chia Seeds—Edible seeds of the *Salvia hispanica* plant that have a high quantity of essential fatty acids. Chia seeds were grown by the Mayan and Aztec cultures and used as a source of energy.

Cleanse Foods—The food groups included in the Paleo Cleanse.

Cleanse Partner—Someone who commits to the Paleo Cleanse with you and helps to hold you accountable.

Coconut Aminos—A great replacement for traditional soy sauce, which is made from fermented soy, coconut aminos are made from raw coconut sap.

Coconut Flour—A Paleo-approved flour that is made from coconut meat.

Coconut Milk—A milk substitute made using coconuts.

Coconut Oil—An oil often used in Paleo cooking and baking. It is made from coconuts and has a low oxidization rate, so is ideal for use at high temperatures.

Cooking Day—The day that you dedicate to cook your meals, either for the whole week or for the next few days.

Cholesterol—A fat-soluble, naturally occurring molecule that can be found in many common foods. Cholesterol comes in two forms: LDL (low-density lipoprotein, commonly known as the "bad" cholesterol) and HDL (high-density lipoprotein, commonly considered to be the "good" cholesterol).

Craving—A strong feeling of wanting something, typically associated with desires for unhealthy foods, i.e., wanting something you shouldn't have.

D-Day—The day you start your Paleo Cleanse.

Evolutionary Biology—The study of evolution among all living organisms through time.

Fiber—A type of carbohydrate that aids the body with digestion. Most often found in fruits and vegetables, fiber is considered the bulky part of food.

The Flintstone Test—Asking yourself "*Would a caveman eat it?*" to help determine if an unknown food is Paleo-friendly or not.

Food as Medicine—The philosophy that eating healthy food leads to overall well-being and can be used to prevent and treat disease.

Food Labels—Labels on food items you purchase; these labels should be read at all times to determine the food's ingredients.

Foods to Avoid at All Costs—The category of food you should not consume during your Paleo Cleanse or on the Paleo Diet.

Free-Range—An environment in which an animal was raised with the ability to roam freely (not to be confused with cage-free).

Fructose—Generally found in honey, fruit, or parts of plants, this simple sugar increases the sugar levels within your body.

Ghee Butter—Butter that has been clarified to help remove some of its fat and dairy content.

Gluten—Protein found in grains, such as wheat, barley, and rye. Shown to negatively affect individuals with gluten sensitivity and celiac disease, gluten also causes digestive complications in a large portion of the population.

Gluten-Free—Foods that do not contain gluten. (Note that this does not always mean that they are also Paleo.)

Glucose—The level of sugar in your bloodstream.

Glyphosate—A herbicide designed to kill weeds, specifically those that compete with commercial crops.

GMO—Also known as a genetically modified organism, or a food that has been genetically modified.

Goji Berry—A fruit of the *Lycium barbarum* plant; considered a superfood, it is rich in protein and minerals.

Grass-Fed—Grass-fed indicates an animal that has lived on a natural diet of grass and is generally leaner and healthier than corn- or grain-fed animals. Grass-fed meat has higher quantities of omega-3 and good cholesterol.

Grocery List—A weekly list we provide to help you shop for the upcoming week of your Cleanse.

Habit—The result of continuously repeating an activity. You'll build new habits and break old ones during your Paleo Cleanse.

Healthy Fats—Fats considered essential to the proper functioning of the human body; found in nuts, oils, and fish.

Healthy Starches—Starches derived from a natural source and which can be digested easily by the human body.

Hormone-Induced Meats—Meats from animals that have been pumped with hormones to make them grow quickly.

Immune System—The body's defense mechanism against foreign entities, which include bacteria and viruses.

Industrial Foods—Foods that are a product of the Industrial Age and are typically mass-produced with preservatives aimed at extending their shelf life unnaturally.

Insulin—A hormone secreted by the pancreas. Insulin helps to process glucose.

Iron—A chemical compound that is critical to the proper function of the human body and aids in red blood cell creation.

Kombucha—A fermented tea that acts as a probiotic.

Lactase Persistent—An individual whose body can digest dairy past early childhood; commonly known as lactose tolerant.

Lactase Non-Persistent—An individual whose body does not process dairy effectively past early childhood; commonly known as lactose intolerant.

Leaky Gut—A condition that occurs as a result of damage to the intestinal wall.

Legume—A legume is a simple dry fruit. The legume family includes peanuts and soy. Legumes are avoided on the Paleo Diet due to the digestive complications they cause.

Maca—A plant native to the mountains of Peru and Bolivia; considered a superfood. Its roots are processed to produce flour that can be incorporated into foods and used for baking and cooking.

Mental Clarity—The ability to focus and maintain a clear train of thought.

Meal Plan—Your plan for what meals you will be eating throughout the week on the Paleo Cleanse.

Meal Plan Options—Your options for meals during each week of the Cleanse.

Natural Energy—Energy that is derived from natural, unprocessed sources.

NBs—Non-Believers. (See Non-Believers)

Nitrate—An ion that is often found in food. Nitrates have been found to have a toxic effect on humans. Nitrates can occur in higher quantities when food is overcooked.

Non-Believers—People who differ in opinion.

Nutrients—Substances with nutritional contents needed for humans to grow and thrive.

Omegas—Fatty acids commonly found in fish and chia seeds; omegas are essential to heart and brain health.

Oxidization—The restructuring of chemical compounds within food that can be triggered during heating; this can cause the food to become toxic.

Pantry Purification—The process of cleaning out your pantry (and other places you store food), ridding them of Paleo-unfriendly food.

Paleo Cleanse—Thirty days of Ancestral eating to detox, drop pounds, supercharge your health, and transition into a primal lifestyle.

Paleo Cleanse Foods—Foods that are included in the Cleanse recipes. You should stock up on these in preparation for your Cleanse.

The Paleo Diet—A diet based on the Paleolithic Era that excludes legumes, wheat, dairy, refined sugars, and processed foods and focuses on the consumption of animal protein, healthy fats, fruits, and vegetables.

Paleo-friendly—A food that is approved for consumption on the Paleo Diet.

Paleo in Moderation—The category of food that you should enjoy in moderation during your Paleo Cleanse.

Paleo Pact—A commitment to being Paleo.

ThePaleoPact.com—Your number-one resource for additional recipes and materials on the Paleo lifestyle (and this isn't because we run it!). Home to the Paleo Cleanse community and bonus online exclusives.

Paleo-unfriendly—A food that is not approved for consumption on the Paleo Diet and during the Cleanse.

Paleolithic Era—(2.6 million years ago to 10,000 B.P.) The era of our ancestors from which the Paleo Diet and Ancestral lifestyle was born.

Primal Diet—A contemporary version of the Ancestral lifestyle that incorporates certain traditionally Paleo-unfriendly foods such as grass-fed dairy; a less strict version of the Paleo Diet.

Probiotic—A substance that contains live bacteria which is used to replace or add to the good bacteria normally present in the stomach.

Protein Powder—A powder that has a large quantity of protein. On the Paleo Diet, egg white protein is largely used as a replacement for traditional protein powders such as whey and soy.

Purchasing Directory—A list of our favorite shopping locations and brands to purchase.

Ramekin—A glazed, ceramic oven dish that can be used for the preparation of food; it is commonly used in our recipes to prepare baked egg dishes.

Refined Sugars—Sugars that have been processed or refined from their original form. These include corn syrup, white sugar, powdered sugar, etc.

Reward Program—A program in which you motive yourself by providing a reward for reaching a set goal.

Sauté Pan—A pan that can be used on a stovetop to cook food, often called a frying pan.

Schools of Paleo—There are several schools of thought that lend themselves to the Paleo Diet; each of them have slight variations based on specific research.

Self-Created Challenge—A challenge that has been imposed on yourself by yourself. They're always the best kind!

Spirulina—A food supplement produced from blue-green algae.

Sugary Fruits—Fruits that have high contents of fructose, such as ripe bananas or melons.

Superfoods—Foods with high phytonutrient contents, believed to provide numerous health benefits.

Tapioca Flour—A starch-based flour derived from the manioc root, often used for Paleo baking and cooking.

Tips—The tips from our own 30-Day Cleanse that we hope will make your journey more successful and enjoyable.

Toxic Proteins—Toxins commonly found in grains and GMOs; these are often referred to as antinutrients.

Truffle Oil—An oil made from olive oil and mushrooms that adds a delicate flavor to dishes.

Veganism—A lifestyle in which you do not consume or use any animal products or by-products.

Vegetarianism—A way of eating in which you do not consume any meat.

Wild-Caught—Fish that has been caught in the wild and was not farmed and has thus lived naturally.

Willpower—That little voice inside your head that says… *You're going to do this and rock it!*

Endnotes

1. Lieberman, Daniel. 2013. "The First Hunter-Gatherers." *The Story of the Human Body: Evolution, Health, and Disease:* 69. New York: Pantheon.

2. Jaminet, Paul, and Shou-Ching Jaminet. 2012. "The Most Toxic Food: Cereal Grains." *Perfect Health Diet: Regain Health and Lose Weight by Eating the Way You Were Meant to Eat:* 197. New York: Scribner.

3. Ibid.

4. Lieberman, Daniel. 2013. "Paradise Lost?" *The Story of the Human Body: Evolution, Health, and Disease:* 206. New York: Pantheon.

5. Cordain, Loren. 2011. *The Paleo Diet: Lose Weight and Get Healthy by Eating the Foods You Were Designed to Eat:* 77. Hoboken, NJ: Wiley.

6. Jaminet, Paul, and Shou-Ching Jaminet. 2012. "Liquid Devils: Vegetable Seed Oils." *Perfect Health Diet: Regain Health and Lose Weight by Eating the Way You Were Meant to Eat:* 217. New York: Scribner.

7. Cordain, Loren. 2011. *The Paleo Diet: Lose Weight and Get Healthy by Eating the Foods You Were Designed to Eat:* 48. Hoboken, NJ: Wiley.

8. "KF Provkök Lanserar Idén Om Basmat." *KF Provkök Lanserar Idén Om Basmat.* http://www.coop.se/Globala-sidor/OmKF/Kooperativ-samverkan/Var historia1/Tidslinjen/1960-19901/1973/KF-Provkok-lanserar-iden-om-basmat/.

9. "Past Food Pyramid Materials," United States Department of Agriculture, http://fnic.nal.usda.gov/dietary-guidance/myplate-and-historical-food-pyramid-resources/past-food-pyramid-materials.

10. "MyPlate & Food Pyramid Resources," Nutrition.gov, http://www.nutrition.gov/smart-nutrition-101/myplate-food-pyramid-resources.

11. Ibid.

12. "Welcome," CrossFit DoneRight, http://cfdrweb.wpengine.netdna-cdn.com/wp-content/uploads/2011/06/paleo_plate.jpg.

13. "Monsanto News, Articles and Information." *NaturalNews.*

14. "Monsanto Bets $5 Million in Fight Over Gene-Altered Food," Bloomberg, http://www.bloomberg.com/news/2013-10-25/monsanto-bets-5-million-in-fight-over-gene-altered-food.html.

15. Jaminet, Paul, and Shou-Ching Jaminet. 2012. "The Most Toxic Food: Cereal Grains." *Perfect Health Diet: Regain Health and Lose Weight by Eating the Way You Were Meant to Eat:* 203–205. New York: Scribner.

16. Ibid., 233.

17. Dur, Jessica, and O. Network. "'Milk Life' Replaces 'Got Milk?' Ad Campaign." *USA Today*, February 24, 2014, http://www.usatoday.com/story/news/nation-now/2014/02/24/got-milk-milk-life-campaign/5776421/.

18. "Also of Interest," National Center for Children in Poverty, http://www.nccp.org/publications/pub_977.html.

19. Jaminet, Paul, and Shou-Ching Jaminet. 2012. "The Most Toxic Foods: Cereal Grains." *Perfect Health Diet: Regain Health and Lose Weight by Eating the Way You Were Meant to Eat:* 199. New York: Scribner.

20. Jaminet, Paul, and Shou-Ching Jaminet. 2012. "Carbohydrates." *Perfect Health Diet: Regain Health and Lose Weight by Eating the Way You Were Meant to Eat:* 91. New York: Scribner.

21. Jaminet, Paul, and Shou-Ching Jaminet. 2012. "Food Toxins Matter." *Perfect Health Diet: Regain Health and Lose Weight by Eating the Way You Were Meant to Eat:* 243. New York: Scribner.

22. Cordain, Loren. 2011. *The Paleo Diet: Lose Weight and Get Healthy by Eating the Foods You Were Designed to Eat:* 38. Hoboken, NJ: Wiley.

23. "The Burden of Skin Diseases," The Society for Investigative Dermatology and the American Academy of Dermatology Association, last modified April 2005, http://www.aad.org/media-resources/stats-and-facts/conditions/acne.

24. "Homepage," *MAGNUM: The National Migraine Association,* http://migraines.org.

25. "Food and Drinks," Migraine.com, http://migraine.com/migraine-triggers/food-and-drinks/.

26. "Brain Fog: Common Causes," Naturopath Connect, http://naturopathconnect.com/articles/brain-fog-causes/.

27. "Sleep Apnea," *American Lung Association.*

28. "Autoimmune Statistics," American Autoimmune Related Diseases Association, Inc., http://www.aarda.org/autoimmune-information/autoimmune-statistics/.

29. Cordain, Loren. 2011. *The Paleo Diet: Lose Weight and Get Healthy by Eating the Foods You Were Designed to Eat:* 93. Hoboken, NJ: Wiley.

30. "Beating Stress Through Nutrition," PsychCentral, http://psychcentral. com/lib/beating-stress-through-nutrition/000941.

31. Jaminet, Paul, and Shou-Ching Jaminet. 2012. "Four Steps to a Low-Toxicity Diet." *Perfect Health Diet: Regain Health and Lose Weight by Eating the Way You Were Meant to Eat*: 236–37. New York: Scribner.

32. Lieberman, Daniel. 2013. "Progress, Mismatch, and Dysevolution." *The Story of the Human Body: Evolution, Health, and Disease:* 168–74. New York: Pantheon.

33. Thompson, R. C., et al. 2013. "Atherosclerosis across 4000 years of human history: The Horus study of four ancient populations." *Lancet. 381*, no. 9873: 1211–22.

34. Jaminet, Paul, and Shou-Ching Jaminet. 2012. "The Safe Fats: SaFA and MUFA." *Perfect Health Diet: Regain Health and Lose Weight by Eating the Way You Were Meant to Eat*: 140. New York: Scribner.

35. "Health Benefits of Grass-Fed Products," EatWild.com, http://www. eatwild.com/healthbenefits.htm.

36. Durant, John. 2013. "Food: The Conventional Wisdom." *The Paleo Manifesto: Ancient Wisdom for Lifelong Health:* 106–107. New York: Harmony.

37. Durant, John. 2013. "Rise and Fall (Paleolithic Age)." *The Paleo Manifesto: Ancient Wisdom for Lifelong Health:* 35–38. New York: Harmony.

38. Li, K., R. Kaaks, J. Linseisen, and S. Rohrmann. 2012. "Associations of Dietary Calcium Intake and Calcium Supplementation with Myocardial Infarction and Stroke Risk and Overall Cardiovascular Mortality in the Heidelberg Cohort of the European Prospective Investigation into Cancer and Nutrition Study (EPIC-Heidelberg)." *Heart* 98, no. 12: 920–25.

39. "Egg Nutrition and Heart Disease," Harvard Health Publications, http:// www.health.harvard.edu/press_releases/egg-nutrition.

40. "Food Allergy Research & Education," Food Allergy Research and Education, http://www.foodallergy.org/allergens.

41. Lieberman, Daniel. 2013 "Paradise Lost?" *The Story of the Human Body: Evolution, Health, and Disease:* 206. New York: Pantheon.

Purchasing Directory

The following is our list of suggestions on where to buy brands we like and foods we have suggested in this book. These items are purely our personal recommendations based on experience and have not been influenced by anything other than that.

In-Person Purchases

The following list of places provides great options for a variety of products. There is a good chance you'll be able to get a hold of almost all (if not every one) of your products at these locations:

Costco: You'll be amazed at what you can find at Costco; some of our favorites to stock up on in bulk are: almond butter, coconut oil, chia seeds, dried fruit, and raw nuts.

Local Butchers or Farmers: They're local and they can generally offer you a great bulk discount; plus, many of them tend to produce organic, grass-fed, free-range products.

Natural Grocers by Vitamin Cottage: You'll find all-natural, high-quality, strictly organic produce—you simply can't go wrong! Plus, you may just catch us hosting a Cooking Demo.

Whole Foods: Great for fresh, grass-fed meat purchases.

Your Local Farmers Market: A wonderful place to find organic vegetables and support the source.

Your Local Grocery Store: You'll be amazed at the products regular grocery stores are now starting to carry to ensure they remain competitive. It's worth taking a look at your local store to see what they now have in stock.

Online Shopping

Wild Mountain Market (www.wildmountainpaleo.com): This store offers a variety of unique Paleo products, including our favorite Paleo coconut wraps.

Brands

The list below showcases brands that we're comfortable with and enjoy a great deal. We recommend trying them out if you haven't already; they are a great place to start:

Beeler's Bacon (www.beelerpurepork.weebly.com): This bacon is fantastic and it's nitrate-free.

Bob's Red Mill (www.bobsredmill.com): The perfect place to purchase bulk Paleo-friendly flours.

Cappello's Pasta (https://cappellosglutenfree.com): This almond flour pasta is premade for you and it's Paleo. We recommend keeping a few of these around for times when you don't feel like cooking. Just make sure you follow the instructions and don't overcook them (they literally cook in under 30 seconds!).

Coconut Secret's Coconut Aminos (www.coconutsecret.com): These aminos are perfect for making teriyaki and Asian-inspired sauces.

Jackson's Honest Sweet Potato Chips (www.honestchips.com): We were so glad to find these sweet potato chips; they're about the only ones that are made with coconut oil and not canola oil.

Justin's Almond Butter, Regular and Honey (www.justins.com): Both of these almond butters pack a great taste, naturally.

MRM, All Natural Egg White Protein Powder (http://mrm-usa. com): Egg white protein powder is the substitute you'll need for traditional soy and dairy-based protein powders; plus, this product is hormone and antibiotic-free.

Navitas Naturals, Cacao Powder (navitasnaturals.com): A certified organic cacao powder that tastes better than chocolate!

Julian Bakery, Paleo Wraps (www.julianbakery.com): These wraps are made strictly from coconut products and are a great alternative to traditional wheat wraps.

Sweet Tree Organic Coconut Palm Sugar (http://bigtreefarms.com): We love to use this sugar for baking; it's particularly great for our Paleo cookies.

Recommended Books & Films

Books

Amsterdam, Elana. *Paleo Cooking from Elana's Pantry: Gluten-free, grain-free, dairy-free recipes*. Ten Speed Press, 2013.

Ballantyne, Sarah. *The Paleo Approach: Reverse autoimmune disease and heal your body*. Victory Belt Publishing, 2014.

Carboni, Camilla, and Melissa Van Dover. *Quick & Fantastic Paleo Cookies*. Camilla Carboni and Melissa Van Dover, 2014. http://thepaleopact.com

Cordain, Loren. *The Paleo Diet: Lose weight and get healthy by eating the foods you were designed to eat*. Houghton Mifflin Harcourt, 2002.

Durant, John, and Michael Malice. *The Paleo Manifesto: Ancient wisdom for lifelong health*. Random House Inc., 2013.

Edwards, Darryl, and Brett Stewart. *Paleo Fitness: Primal training and nutrition to get lean, strong and healthy*. Ulysses Press, 2013.

Lieberman, Daniel. *The Story of the Human Body: Evolution, health, and disease*. Pantheon, 2013.

Robinson, Jo. *Eating on the Wild Side: The missing link to optimum health*. Little, Brown and Company, 2013.

Tam, Michelle, and Henry Fong. *Nom Nom Paleo: Food for humans*. Andrews McMeel Publishing, 2013.

Films

Food, Inc. Directed by Robert Kenner. Magnolia Pictures, 2008.

The Perfect Human Diet. Directed by C. J. Hunt. Passion River Films, 2013.

Conversions

USEFUL CONVERSIONS

U.S. MEASURE	EQUIVALENT	METRIC
1 teaspoon	—	5 milliliters
1 tablespoon	3 teaspoons	15 milliliters
1 cup	16 tablespoons	240 milliliters
1 pint	2 cups	470 milliliters
1 quart	4 cups	950 milliliters
1 liter	4 cups + 3½ tablespoons	1000 milliliters
1 ounce (dry)	2 tablespoons	28 grams
1 pound	16 ounces	450 grams
2.21 pounds	35.3 ounces	1 kilogram
270°F / 350°F	—	132°C / 177°C

VOLUME CONVERSIONS

U.S. MEASURE	EQUIVALENT	METRIC
1 tablespoon	½ fluid ounce	15 milliliters
¼ cup	2 fluid ounces	60 milliliters
⅓ cup	3 fluid ounces	90 milliliters
½ cup	4 fluid ounces	120 milliliters
⅔ cup	5 fluid ounces	150 milliliters
¾ cup	6 fluid ounces	180 milliliters
1 cup	8 fluid ounces	240 milliliters
2 cups	16 fluid ounces	480 milliliters

WEIGHT CONVERSIONS

U.S. MEASURE	METRIC
1 ounce	30 grams
⅓ pound	150 grams
½ pound	225 grams
1 pound	450 grams

Index

Acknowledgments

Without the support of each other and those closest to us, our own Paleo challenge would have been a lot more challenging and this book might never have been written. Thank you also to those who challenged us—you made us stronger, more educated and more pumped than before. We love you all!

Many thanks to our Beta Readers for your time and your insight.

Thank you to Kelly Reed and the whole Ulysses Press team for believing in us and bringing this book to life. We are forever grateful.

Camilla Carboni and Melissa Van Dover

To my boyfriend, Matt, for introducing me to the Paleo Diet and for encouraging me to begin this Paleo journey—you have made the experience incredible. Thank you for equipping us with recipe books, researching the best places to purchase organic, grass-fed meats and bulk quantities of coconut flour, sharing many evenings with me experimenting in our kitchen, and saying that my half-risen Paleo desserts still tasted delicious. You're the best!

To my mom, Joan, for teaching me the importance of being healthy, showing me the potential in life, instilling in me a go-getter attitude, and always believing in me and encouraging me to write. None of this would have ever come about without you. You are the most incredible inspiration and the world's best supporter.

To my cat, Bruce, for relentlessly sitting on my lap as I wrote—you are my silent partner.

To my angels—Daps, Gran, Pegs, and Denise—these words were written with you in mind.

Love you all, Camilla

To my husband, Ryan. How you put up with my craziness in general I'll never know. Thank you for letting me spend all my time writing and for being my guinea pig during the testing of all my Paleo dishes. I was able to tell with certainty if a dish was good depending upon whether or not I could actually get you to eat it.

To my parents. Mom and Dad, thank you for teaching me that life is what you make it and that I can live my dreams if I'm willing to fight for them hard enough. You've supported me through everything—even my first try at Paleo brownies, when you ate the entire dish (by the way, I know they really weren't that good).

To my brother, Matt: Here's to following our dreams, making big things happen, and changing the world.

Love you always, Melissa

About the Authors

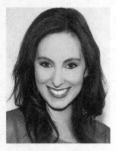

Camilla Carboni is the co-founder of *The Paleo Pact* and co-author of *Quick & Fantastic Paleo Cookies*. Camilla applies her global marketing portfolio and Master's in Media Reception Psychology to promote the philosophy of health from the inside out. Camilla is a South African expat, minimalist runner, and contributor to various lifestyle publications. She lives her American Dream in Colorado with her supportive boyfriend and adoring cat.

Learn more at CamillaCarboni.com.

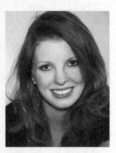

Melissa Van Dover is the co-founder of *The Paleo Pact* and co-author of *Quick & Fantastic Paleo Cookies*. Melissa utilizes her marketing background and MBA to promote the importance of maintaining a healthy lifestyle through eating well and regular exercise. Melissa currently resides in Colorado, where she spends her time practicing Pilates and enjoying the outdoors with her loving husband.

Learn more at MelissaVanDover.com.

The Paleo Pact is dedicated to assisting others in beginning and sustaining their Paleo journey toward optimum health. Visit ThePaleoPact.com for free recipes and resources throughout your Paleo Cleanse and beyond.